T0130774

MISUNDERSTANDING HEALTH

MISUNDERSTANDING
HEALTH

MAKING SENSE OF AMERICA'S BROKEN HEALTH CARE SYSTEM

Rohit Khanna

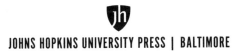
JOHNS HOPKINS UNIVERSITY PRESS | BALTIMORE

Johns Hopkins University Press
2715 North Charles Street
Baltimore, Maryland 21218-4363
www.press.jhu.edu

Library of Congress Cataloging-in-Publication Data

Names: Khanna, Rohit, 1968– author.
Title: Misunderstanding Health : Making Sense of America's Broken
Health Care System / Rohit Khanna.
Description: Baltimore : Johns Hopkins University Press, 2021. |
Includes bibliographical references and index.
Identifiers: LCCN 2020056261 | ISBN 9781421442099 (hardcover : alk. paper) |
ISBN 9781421442105 (ebook)
Subjects: MESH: Delivery of Health Care | Health Policy |
Social Determinants of Health | Health Behavior | United States | Popular Work
Classification: LCC RA425 | NLM W 84 AA1 | DDC 362.1—dc23
LC record available at https://lccn.loc.gov/2020056261

A catalog record for this book is available from the British Library.

*Special discounts are available for bulk purchases of this book. For more information, please
contact Special Sales at specialsales@jh.edu.*

CONTENTS

MISUNDERSTANDING
HEALTH

Introduction

सत्यमेवजयते [Truth alone triumphs.]
—A mantra from the ancient Indian scripture *Mundaka Upanishad*. After India's independence, it was adopted as the national motto. It is inscribed in script at the base of the national emblem.

In February 2017, one of the greatest one-liners in modern times was uttered when the forty-fifth president of the United States stood at a podium in the White House and said, "Nobody knew that health care could be so complicated." Actually, we did Mr. President. Or, at least, most of us did. That pronouncement was so ridiculous on its face that I actually went to one of those websites that allows you to print business cards, flyers, posters, and other paraphernalia and had a T-shirt made with that quote on the back. My fear was that the internet would one day be extinguished, and we would have no record of this outlandish statement. With said T-shirt safely tucked into a drawer in my closet, I now felt strangely secure that future generations would not be able to challenge the veracity of the statement. "I mean, it's on a T-shirt!" I would proclaim.

That health care has *always* been complex is a given, despite what some duly elected officials have opined. That health care's complexity is *more complex* than previously thought is, perhaps, a novel idea. It is revealing that even the most well informed of us who spend our time on health policy, health economics, and public health and who are at the front lines of treating and caring for patients and who are in the darkened laboratories looking for new molecules to treat today's deadliest diseases did not appreciate how complex health care was and how it continues to be ever more complex, day in and day out.

That the degree of health care's complexity is not fixed is something that I've been aware of for years. And that is not a good thing. Pricing and drug development are becoming more, not less, complex. New diseases and fancy biologic and precision medicine therapies are at a higher order of complexity than we had, say, a generation or two ago. Access to health care could have been easier and more transparent thanks to technological advances; instead, it's become muddled with the advent of all this wonderful technology. A dizzying array of health insurance options have multiplied from yesteryear. And the list goes on. My long view of health care at the turn of the twenty-first century was that innovation and technology would usher in an era of simplification and adroitness that would make things easier.

Health care is not complex. It's *more* complex than it has been in the past. And that's what I want you to take away from this book. Not in a depressing sort of way, like the way we look at the calculus problem on our grade 10 final exam and think it's unsolvable. But in the way that implores, "Hey, it's OK. Let's all get comfortable with this because we can get a handle on it, and it's not out of reach."

I dearly want readers also to understand and embrace, beyond the obvious complexity of health care, the idea that our behavior and our everyday decisions—both in the comfort of our own homes and in the corridors of our state legislatures—can greatly influence almost everything about health care. The great behavioral thinkers of our time from Kahneman to Thaler to Gladwell to Levitt have elucidated this concept beautifully over the past two decades, both in an academic and a practical setting. Whether it's the doctrine of nudges or freakonomics, we are more cognizant of how our own individual behavior and, indeed, the collective behavior along with incentives shape our actual health and our health policies.

So, within this context of a complex subject that hinges on the vagaries and nuances of individual and societal behavior, I have written eighteen essays. Each essay is its own sketch of a topic that is, in my view, critical to better understanding the present-day complexities of health care. While there is some calculated and purposeful overlap between the essays and their topics, the stark differences among the topics is also intentional. Because, as actors within the larger health care ecosystem, we are also all different. Therefore, our experience with health and health care—which shapes our viewpoint and perspective—is naturally different, too. I hope, in reading these essays, that you recognize an experience somewhere in these pages.

1

All the King's Men

The end of man is knowledge, but there is one thing he can't know. He can't know whether knowledge will save him or kill him. He will be killed, all right, but he can't know whether he is killed because of the knowledge which he has got or because of the knowledge which he hasn't got and which if he had it, would save him.   —ROBERT PENN WARREN, *All the King's Men*

Imagine if you were Martin Shkreli. Not the being sent to prison part. Not the buying a rare $2 million Wu-Tang Clan album part either. But the part where you were easily one of the top ten most hated businesspeople in the country for three years running. Now imagine that everyone in the country also owed you a collective thank-you. It's a rare occurrence indeed that someone can be so repulsive, yet we are so much in his debt for the light he has shone on an issue.

Shkreli is not alone. We can thank Heather Bresch, Brent Saunders, and, while we're at it, Gilead Pharmaceuticals as well. And countless others.

Let's be clear, we have known for decades that pharma prices made no sense. Professor Uwe Reinhardt of Princeton University and Professor Gerard Anderson of Johns Hopkins University told us as much in their landmark article "It's the Prices, Stupid," published in 2003, which looked at the latest data from the Organisation for Economic Co-operation and Development to compare the health systems of the thirty member countries in 2000. The results: the United States spends more on health care than any other country. On most measures of health services use, however, the United States is below the OECD median. The authors suggest that the spending difference is because of variations in the prices of goods and services among countries.[1]

Despite this landmark academic article, nothing has ever happened. We could smell the rank odor of the pricing process, and we were able to bear witness to the ludicrous verbal gymnastics of those who attempted to explain the process, but the outrageous prices continued. Prices were there but not really there. We thought about these things. It wasn't the type of thing that we spoke about but rather the stuff of policy wonks and health economists who mixed in "those" circles. We complained, and we grumbled. But like our grousing about bank fees and the price of gas, it got lost in the noise and the never-ending conversation of how everything in life had gotten *so* expensive.

Then September 2015 happened. Martin Shkreli and Turing Pharmaceuticals obtained the manufacturing license for the antiparasitic drug Daraprim and raised its price by a factor of 56 (from US$13.50 to $750 per pill).[2] Only two thousand Americans use Daraprim every year. And while toxoplasmosis affects an estimated 22.5 percent of Americans over the age of twelve, typically only people with immune systems weakened by HIV/AIDS, cancer treatment, organ transplants, or pregnancy need the medication.[3] To dismiss these small numbers relative to some larger and more common diseases such as cardiovascular disease, diabetes, and respiratory illnesses would be to miss the point. The world gasped. How could he? Hands started wringing everywhere. Talk shows and social media platforms were abuzz. No less than presidential candidate Hillary Clinton tweeted out about it and promised to address price gouging in the pharmaceutical industry.[4]

And because of this buzz, as Malcolm Gladwell would surely tell us, the tipping point had just occurred—"the moment of critical mass, the threshold, the boiling point."[5] It didn't take a major *60 Minutes* exposé or some hard-hitting undercover journalism from the *New York Times*. It didn't take dying patients toting placards in the streets. It took internet outrage. It took normal, decent people to understand that taking advantage of the most vulnerable in our society is just wrong. And, thus, the tipping point that Gladwell had introduced us to became instantly recognizable.

And then came the EpiPen con job. Mylan pharmaceuticals raised the price of the EpiPen from $100 in 2004 to over $600 in 2016 (figure 1). Decidedly unapologetic as she testified before Congress, Mylan CEO Heather Bresch attempted to deflect much of the blame to the system of intermediaries and their thirst for profit.[6] The EpiPen, for those who may not remember, is a device that delivers the drug epinephrine, which is a lifesaving medication used when someone is experiencing a severe allergic reaction, known as anaphylaxis.[7] And by some estimates, more than 3.6 million Americans used the device in 2015.[8]

Of course, who among us can forget the cheeky "let's transfer our patent to an American Indian tribe" schtick that Brent Saunders pulled for Allergan and its lead drug, Restasis. Restasis is basically used for the treatment of chronic dry eye and to increase tear production in patients who may be compromised because of ocular inflammation.[9] In 2015, there were 1.57 million Medicare claims for Restasis.[10] The ironically funny thing about this Restasis story is that we're genuinely not even sure that this drug works. In a recent

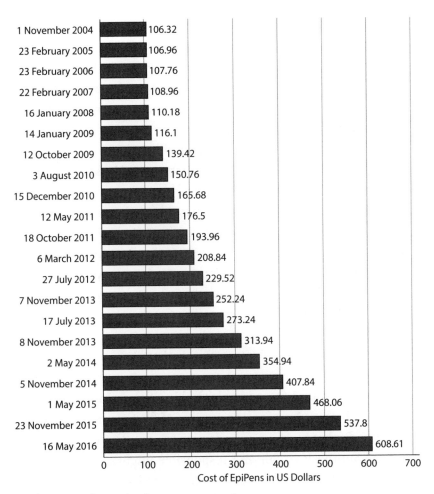

Figure 1. EpiPen price from 2004 to 2016.

JAMA Internal Medicine article published in 2018, two researchers from the Center for Medicine in the Media at the Dartmouth Institute for Health Policy and Clinical Practice looked at this fundamental question and made the case that Restasis was approved on the basis of very weak evidence.[11] They went on to point out that Restasis was denied approval in Australia and New Zealand on the basis of the same evidence package, that it is currently not approved in Europe, and that Canada's cost-effectiveness watchdogs have been wholly unconvinced of the drug's benefits and will not allow it to be paid for by the government.[12] But I digress.

In fairness to Saunders, the evidence package for Restasis and its lack of regulatory approval almost everywhere else in the world predates his arrival at Allergan. Nonetheless, protection of the golden goose was of utmost importance. So, here's what Saunders and his brain trust thought: let's find a willing dance partner, immune from federal oversight in such matters, and let's transfer our product's patents to them to free ourselves of the numerous court challenges that we face that threaten to encroach on our commercial exclusivity. You see, American Indian tribes, along with institutions such as universities, have sovereign immunity that protects patents from certain challenges to their validity; so, the two sides struck a deal that would give the Saint Regis Mohawk Tribe an up-front payment of $13.75 million with an annual royalty stream of $15 million.[13]

This deal was done *after* Saunders had made a social contract with patients, posting it for everyone to see.[14] In this contract, Saunders promised fair and responsible pricing along with "facilitating better access to our medicines."[15] Lost in this entire narrative is that blocking generic entry and stifling competition are the antithesis of fair and responsible pricing. By doing so, the system overpays for medications for millions of people for years and years. Saunders and his team argued that the industry was sick of inter partes reviews that challenged product patents and gave generic companies an easy backdoor into commercializing soon-to-expire molecules. It didn't go very well. The Patent Trial and Appeal Board struck down Allergan's attempt to conduct an end run around the system and ruled that the Saint Regis Mohawk Tribe could not use its sovereign immunity status for such purposes.

Last, Gilead, the drug company that brought us Sovaldi, the hepatitis C medication that costs $1,000 a pill. The drug company that threatened to bankrupt entire state-level Medicaid programs because of its pricing and the number of patients who benefited from the drug. In the United States, the estimated prevalence of chronic HCV infection was 2.7 million, based on survey data from 2003 to 2010; however, this estimate probably understated the true prevalence because the survey excluded key high-risk populations, such as homeless and incarcerated individuals.[16] The Centers for Disease Control and Prevention currently estimates the number of chronically infected people in the United States at 2.7 million to 3.9 million.[17] At a Brookings Institution panel discussion entitled, "The Cost and Value of Biomedical Innovation: Implications for Health Policy," Gilead CEO John Milligan stated that "it was ultimately the prices of previous therapies that determined their approach to price. He acknowledged that while they believe Sovaldi has a return on investment (ROI), Gilead did not attempt to factor ROI into any consideration of the price—it was simply looking at the previous, less desirable therapy and going up from there."[18] Gilead then launched a follow-on combination pill to Sovaldi that was even more expensive than the original one.

What are the lessons from this narrative? There are many, but there are three key ones, each from a different stakeholder viewpoint: legislators, patients, and drug manufacturers.

The first lesson is that drug companies are largely unchecked in their ability to charge whatever they want for their products in the United States. Yes, states can try to impose mechanisms to limit drug company price increases, to provide advance notice of price increases, or to justify price increases before implementing them, including through legislation. To date, more than 150 bills to rein in prescription drug costs have been introduced or approved in state legislatures across the country.[19] But the drug companies can challenge legislation—as they have done in California where the drug price transparency law, known as SB 17, was challenged by PhRMA (the country's leading lobby group on behalf of innovative pharmaceutical companies) on various constitutional grounds. Or as they have done in Maryland. Or Nevada. And maybe the courts will rule that these price transparency laws are legally binding. Or they won't. And then we're right back where we started.

Maybe states can try something that doesn't mandate that companies reveal their pricing strategy: How about a money-back guarantee? The state's position is this: If we buy your drug and your drug doesn't work, then we want our money back. It's called value-based pricing, and, to be fair, it has some merit. The health care industry might be the only industry vertical in which there is no mechanism for a refund for the consumer if a product doesn't work. Value-based pricing attempts to change that. But when a drug company returns money to a state's coffers, we are still left with sick people. It seems obvious, but we often forget that, if a state purchases a medication that promises a certain outcome and doesn't deliver on that outcome, we are no better off. In fact, we may be worse off. Patients may have been treated with a medication that provided no benefit and that allowed their disease to progress such that different interventions are now required or additional diagnostics and clinical services are needed. Patients with arthritis try expensive biologic drugs at a cost of tens of thousands of dollars per year, and sometimes these therapies don't work. Sometimes, patients are left with worsened joint disease. More tender joints. More swollen joints. More joint erosion. A reduced quality of life.

So, while we cheer and pat ourselves on the back for getting our money back, we are left with thousands (millions, even?) of patients who still have unmanaged disease, who still occupy hospital beds, and who still draw upon our finite resources. We should understand that value-based pricing is meant to serve as the framework for a larger idea. We all understand that a refund model will not be perfect. We all understand that some buyers (patients) will get refunds when they shouldn't, and others will not get refunds when they should. We all understand that we can come up with at least ten outlier scenarios that poke holes in this refund model. But here's the upshot: with new therapies that cost upward of $14,000 per year to treat high cholesterol, such as Praluent or Repatha, and therapies that cost six figures to treat cancers and rare diseases, the model *has* to change.

We can no longer afford to simply shrug our shoulders when treatments don't work and continue to pay for them. I don't think manufacturers would want us to either since the future viability and reimbursement of their drugs, both private and public, depend on the system's ability to pay for today's drugs. If we overpay today, we lose the ability to pay tomorrow. We need a starting point—no matter how imperfect—that strives to balance the cost burden between those who benefit, those who pay, and those who produce. The Italians have a system like this. The Italian Medicines Agency has devised deals with pharma companies that set payments based on how well a patient responds to treatment, and, in some cases, where the medication fails to help, the drug maker gives a full refund. The medicines agency—responsible for drug regulation in Italy—established national registries in 2005 that track all patients' treatments and their outcomes, which provide the basis for the assessments and allow the agency to renegotiate contracts based on new data every two years or so. We're not talking about a handful of products or an insignificant amount of money either. Italy was able to get approximately €200 million of a rebate—representing 1 percent of its national health budget—on utilization of over ninety different medications. Italy seems to be so smitten with this approach that it has more than quadrupled the number of treatments under this innovative risk-sharing scheme (figure 2).[20]

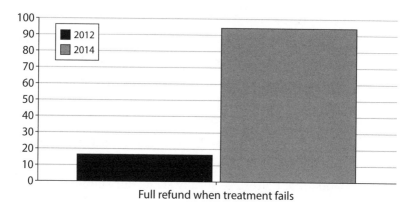

Figure 2. Number of drugs in Italy where a full refund is given if treatment fails.

The second lesson is that, at the macro level, people care about drug costs and fancy terms such as *cost-effectiveness* and *quality adjusted life years*, or QALYs. Policy makers and budget holders fret over the rising costs, forcing us to make enormously difficult trade-off decisions, such as who should get priority over these new expensive medications or whether the medications should even be reimbursed in the first place. Perhaps we even worry at our soccer games and dinner parties, but that is window-dressing worry. At the real micro level—the level of the individual patient and family—we ignore these prices. Not because we want to. Because we are forced to. If you're too poor to afford health care or have no insurance, what difference does an extra zero make on your drug costs? You can't afford $500 per month, nor can you afford $5,000. And if you're middle class, you probably have a middle-class job with middle-class insurance. Your employer-based insurance covers some of your drug costs, and you cover the rest. Sure, you're approaching your annual cap or your lifetime cap, but you have to keep working to pay for the drugs that your employer plan doesn't cover. And, well, if you're rich, then you don't have to worry because you can pay for your drugs without batting an eyelid. An oversimplification? Of course, it is. But not far from reality. Therefore, the upshot of the second lesson is that as disaggregated individuals—dare I say, data points—we have to find a way to pay for our drugs or ration our prescriptions so that our supply lasts or rely on government aid and funding wherever it may exist. Someone, at the macro level, worries about everyone. At the micro level, we worry about no one but ourselves.

The third lesson that we learn from this narrative of drug price raising is grounded partly in the behavioral sciences and partly in the consumer world of advertising: to raise prices, you must justify them. You must give me more horsepower or better gas mileage. You must give me a ten-megapixel camera instead of an eight-megapixel or more storage or a longer battery life. Tell me *why* you're raising your price. Or better yet, tell me what *more* I'm getting for this increased price. This is where the pharmaceutical industry has fallen flat on its face. Both patented and generic companies have become so used to making annual price increases that in many cases there is no justification for it. A price increase that mirrors the inflation rate or the consumer price index would be easy to understand. But no one understands double- to triple-digit price increases over twenty-four to thirty-six months. It does not compute. Either you are totally inept at running your company and are unable to understand the production costs that go into making your product, which is why you can't get a handle on your pricing and need to constantly raise it, or you are greedy and see an opportunity to make money off the backs of needy, sick people. Or both. But when you invoke trade secrets, use constitutional amendments as part of your argument, and generally challenge price-transparency laws at every chance you get, people smell a rat.

Remember, when you cite research and development costs as the reason your drugs are so expensive, that argument only works for the drug's *initial* price. It does not explain why you must keep raising the price every single year. Repeating the "R&D costs have to be recouped" mantra suggests an echo chamber mentality. Saying that you run a publicly traded company that is responsible to its shareholders grossly oversimplifies the issue that most people don't care to listen to. When companies tweak the formulation of their product to extend the patent life, it is disingenuous. Reformulating drugs adds years to system costs by delaying the entry of generic drugs that, in the aggregate, can save millions of dollars per year. When Lilly faced the expiration of its patent for the blockbuster antidepressant drug Prozac, the company developed and obtained patent protection and US Food and Drug Administration approval for a once-weekly, sustained-release fluoxetine formulation—a cosmetic change that the company could have made available at launch or soon thereafter. Bristol Myers Squibb also did essentially the same thing for its extended-release formulation of the diabetes drug Glucophage by marketing it under its new brand name, Glucophage XR.[21] None of these examples can justify egregious price increases.

We are forever different post–Martin Shkreli than we were before. That is not an exaggeration. Every shameless attempt to increase prices now receives stunningly thorough media attention. This was not the case five years ago. Or ten. Or twenty. But the problem is that the behavior of drug companies hasn't changed. And it isn't just the behavior of the drug companies. It's the pharmacy benefits managers and the insurance companies, too. We've become immune to it all because a drug's cost only matters when you need medicine. When you're healthy, you pay attention to drug prices as much as you pay attention to the unemployment rate when you have a job. When you need the medicine, you don't have time to worry about the cost. You only have time to worry about getting well. We are outraged for a few moments, and then we turn our attention to other matters. Hundreds of solutions have been put forward and some have serious potential. But what we know is that there is no one single solution and that every time we plug one hole, another one opens up. In the end, we are immensely thankful to the Martin Shkrelis of the world. We are not thankful because they shine a light on themselves and others in the industry that they truly had no intention of doing. We *know* they would have preferred to continue on in anonymity without drawing more attention to themselves than necessary. We are thankful because their actions remind us that, to paraphrase George Orwell, it is the first duty of intelligent men everywhere to pay attention to the obvious. What is sometimes obvious is how we react to attempts to remove the very foundations of health care that we have come to rely on.

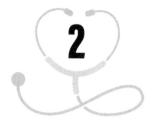

Heads I Win, Tails You Lose

At the temple there is a poem called "Loss" carved into the stone. It has three words, but the poet has scratched them out. You cannot read loss, only feel it.
—ARTHUR GOLDEN, *Memoirs of a Geisha*

It's hard to take something away once you've given it to someone, let alone tens of millions of people. It's even harder to take away something when you have no backup plan to replace the very thing you're planning on taking away with something new. Not better. Just new. Different. Anything. But not nothing. Nothing is the worst thing you could replace this something with.

Republicans in the United States expended monumental effort to repeal and replace the Affordable Care Act (ACA)—President Barack Obama's landmark health care bill from 2010, which strove, among many things, to reduce total health system costs, to increase access to care and services, and to provide Americans with the type of coverage that would eliminate discrimination based on preexisting conditions. A large part of Republicans' reasoning, as articulated by House Speaker Paul Ryan, was that "government shouldn't be [this] involved in people's healthcare." It comes back to the party's notion that the role of government is to follow the path of least intrusion. However, for those of us who believe in the principles of behavioral economics, this is folly. Behavioral economics studies the effects of psychological, social, cognitive, and emotional factors on the economic decisions of individuals and institutions and the consequences for market prices, returns, and resource allocation. The health and social policy literature are littered with examples of people needing nudges and of social experiments where we see clearly that individual decision making is shaky and tenuous. You may view these nudges and social experiments as government overreach. That is your prerogative. However you view them, it is more important perhaps that you accept that they exist and that they are here to stay, not as a means of intruding in your life but as a means of social equality. Many people can't make decisions; they need help. They need to be pointed in the right direction explicitly or by an invisible hand.

The debate about the ACA, also called Obamacare, offered some important lessons. First, it's not easy to make Obamacare, which accounts for 20 percent of total gross domestic product, just go away, backup plan or not. But it's also true of the individual elements and clauses within the act. Preexisting conditions? Don't you dare touch that! Children covered on their parents' plan until the age of twenty-six? Absolutely, we need it. Federally established essential health benefits and services? Unequivocally, yes. Thus, even if you try and chop it up into smaller pieces, it's hard to take away. Why? Because big pieces of legislation are inextricably linked by smaller parts of the whole. Like a trusted recipe for your favorite dish, when a smaller part of the whole is taken away, it leaves a bad taste.

The behavioral sciences have taught us for decades that taking things away elicits a very strong reaction in people. Loss aversion is what we call it. And empirical studies have shown that it's about twice as powerful psychologically as the prospect of gaining something.[1] Those same behavioral sciences have also taught us that language and words can be critically important drivers of behavior. It's both remarkable and bizarre that a president who has used psychology and communication as effectively as, if not better than, anyone else who has occupied the Oval Office missed this one. Or, equally likely, perhaps, everyone told him to stay away from those two words (repeal and replace), but he chose not to listen.

If Republicans were to have succeeded in this Obamacare exercise, it is clear to me that the focus needed to be on building and improving instead of repealing and replacing. This failed policy shift is as much a lesson in communication and the subtlety of language and word choice as it is about navigating the corridors of power, working in a bipartisan manner, and astute health policy. By articulating words such as *repeal* and *replace*, there is a palpable sense of a void and a hole and with it an inescapable connotation: that repealing and replacing implies *I must give something up. I am going to lose something.*

Are you skeptical that different words could have influenced this debacle that was the Republican strategy? Look at figure 3 and ask whether countries represented by the cluster of shorter histograms and taller histograms were influenced by word choice.[2] You see, the difference in organ donation rates between the first four countries (represented by the shorter histograms) and the last seven countries (represented by the taller histograms) is not a consequence of a more caring society, efficient government planning and implementation regarding organ donation, or some set of austere and mandatory laws for driver's license renewal. The difference, almost exclusively, boils down to the choice of words used on people's driver license applications and renewals and how these words frame decisions (figure 4). If you want people to donate, make donating the default option. Make people do something (like tick a box) and take some action to get out of donating. This is not a commentary on people's laziness. This shows that when people have to make complex decisions they sometimes choose to do nothing. Remember that when you opt out of something, the individual perspective is, again, of loss. Opting out implies that you're currently already in. And if you're currently in, then to opt out would be to *give something up*. Why do I go out of my way to mention this example that has nothing to do with repealing and replacing Obamacare? Because it reinforces the point

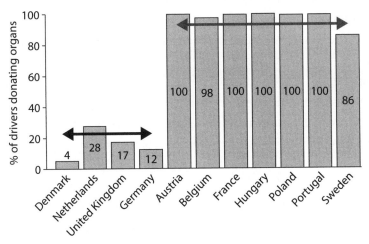

Figure 3. Organ donations in select European countries.

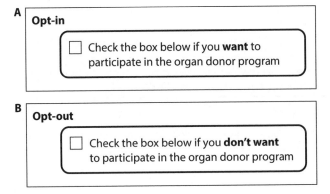

Figure 4. *A,* Question asked on driver's license applications and renewals in shorter histogram countries. *B,* Question asked on driver's license applications and renewals in taller histogram countries.

that words, language, and how choices and decisions are framed matter when you talk to people about health care.

Loss aversion in health care has been a concern for decades. Before Obamacare became the law of the land and while it was being hotly debated, we knew then, too, that loss aversion in health care was a political hot potato. A survey experiment in 2009, amid the debate over health care reform, illustrates loss aversion within the context of health insurance.[3] Respondents to this survey were randomly assigned to one of two different groups and then asked to make a hypothetical choice between two optional health care plans (table 1). The percentages in the table represent the proportion of respondents who chose a particular option depending on which group they were in. In both cases, the absence of a lifetime limit on health insurance benefits would cost the respondent $1,000 per year. In group 1, the cost would come because the respondent didn't choose the plan that could have saved money, which is what almost 80 percent of people did. In group 2, the cost is directly tied to the lifetime limit. However, despite the equivalence, the different framing of the options (one emphasizing savings, the other focusing on cost) is critical.[4] This example demonstrates what we have always known (except for a few Republicans in the United States apparently): framing choices

Table 1. Fictitious scenario of two optional health plans

Question: Suppose you were offered a choice between the following two health insurance plans. Which one would you choose?

	Group 1	Group 2
Option 1	A plan with no lifetime limit on benefits. (79.5%)	A plan that limited the total amount of benefits in your lifetime to $1 million. (44.2%)
Option 2	A plan that limited the total amount of benefits in your lifetime to $1 million but saved you $1,000 per year. (20.5%)	A plan with no lifetime limit on benefits but cost you an additional $1,000 per year. (55.8%)

and the presentation of such choices as costs versus savings can greatly affect perceptions and behavior in health care.

Another lesson from this failed Republican effort shows that people do not always make health care decisions in their own best interest; in some instances, they don't even make better decisions than someone else can make on their behalf. Conventional examples help to illustrate this concept: people still smoke, lead sedentary lives with minimal exercise, consume diets rich in fats and added sugars, and refuse to get vaccinated despite the obvious benefits of herd immunity. On their own, let alone collectively, each of these behaviors is clearly not in the best interest of the individual. Other people—a clinician or a loved one, for example—could make a better decision for the individual concerned.

However, the mistaken idea that people are the best judges of their own health remains a tenet of our approach to health care, and it helps explain the debate. People make bad decisions. This is not an exhortation for extreme government involvement in all aspects of health care; it is an acknowledgment that, intentionally or unintentionally, countries that have some level of essential benefits and services set out by the government may be onto something. Those countries may have figured out (or blindly stumbled on) that, if we give people a basic basket of essential health services, it eliminates complexity and might lead to better overall outcomes at a population level. We need to accept that people bring biases to decision making and that those biases may be a function of many things, including one's inability to understand what they are being told.

The third lesson from the raging debate that engulfs the American health care system manifests itself in the individual mandate. This is the aspect of the ACA that, until January 2019, required individuals to either purchase health insurance or face a penalty if they didn't. Part of this ACA clause is rooted in the theory of expected utility, which examines how people make decisions under conditions of uncertainty. The basic principle is that, when faced with a choice of something certain or the gamble or trade-off of an uncertain outcome between two options, there will be a point of neutrality or, to be blunt, a point of indifference. With this backdrop in mind, Obamacare attempted to establish this point of indifference that might motivate healthy people to buy insurance, which would help premiums stay within an affordable range. Here's what happened with Obamacare's individual mandate in a nutshell: healthy people were mandated to buy health insurance, and they did (sometimes very grudgingly). Sick and vulnerable people also bought health insurance (also, believe it or not, grudgingly). The risk pool now had lots of healthy people and a fair number of sick people. Insurance companies were happy, as they collected premiums from the entire risk pool and only paid out to those who were sick and made claims. Premiums stayed relatively stable in this scenario. But, if healthy people were released from the onus of having to buy health insurance by, say, some court ruling that stipulated this individual mandate were no longer necessary, well, that would be a different story

In this scenario, those same risk pools would now have an exodus of healthy members. The healthy members would no longer be required to keep paying premiums for a policy that they never made any claims against. But the risk pools would still retain their sick members. Now, the insurance companies would start paying out claims at a higher rate than the premiums they were collecting because everyone in their risk membership pool was less than healthy. They would raise premiums the following year to offset their anticipated losses for having to cover so many sick people. And when they raised rates, the sick people wouldn't be able to afford their new insurance policy, so they would exit the risk pool, too, and go without insurance. This cycle would repeat itself over and over again in thousands of miniature risk pools all over America. And while the individual mandate of the ACA was repealed in January 2019, it remains to be seen whether the mass exodus of the healthy insured actually happens and whether it destabilizes the insurance marketplace.

In health economics, we have what we call indifference curves (figure 5); we define this phenomenon as the scenario in which a consumer's utility, or preference, between two goods is of equal value. That is to say that the consumer has no preference for one combination or bundle of goods over a different combination on the same curve. In other words, there is a point at which health care consumers ought to be indifferent about buying insurance and paying a penalty if they don't. The trick is to harness this indifference such that they do buy the insurance. This is no easy feat. There is no blueprint for how to do this. The irony is obvious. In the field of medicine and public health, we are taught from our early days to focus on caring and treating people with respect and dignity. Instead, sometimes not caring—being, in fact, indifferent—just might be the most powerful lesson of them all.

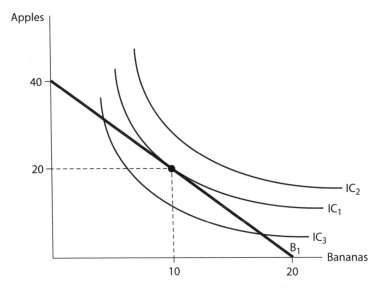

Figure 5. Sample indifference curve showing the varying levels of two commodities.

The great martial artist and philosopher Bruce Lee said this of water: "When you pour water in a cup, it becomes the cup. When you pour water in a bottle, it becomes the bottle. When you pour water in a teapot, it becomes the teapot." Health care is like water. A nation's identity is the cup. Health care becomes the embodiment of a nation. This is our fourth lesson. To truly "fix" health care, it must embody your nation. It must be a part of who you are. In many countries, people speak with pride about their commitment to a social system that relies and insists on the premise that I will look after you when you are old and that the next generation will look after me when I am old. It is this pay-it-forward mentality that makes health care go. In Canada, where I live, health care, with all its imperfections, has become an integral part of our identities. This is not just a Canadian thing. When you travel to Europe and speak with the English, the French, the Germans, the Swiss, it becomes immediately obvious that other countries, too, have allowed health care to shape their national identities. In America, this phenomenon has not occurred. Health care is, in some respects, regarded as an enemy. A suspicious intruder that is here to rob us of our hard-earned dollars and that answers to private corporate entities that do not have our best interests at heart. How the nation organizes its health care system has never been an intrinsic part of what it means to be American. Because of this, it feels like it's easier for Americans to discard it (or parts of it) with the arrival of every new administration.

And so, in the end, the American system seems to be caught in an echo chamber of sound bites emanating from two political parties whose views on health care are so fundamentally different. The lessons we learn do not stop with loss aversion. Social and public health policy do not afford us the luxury of thinking about the individuality of health care. We cannot think of the "ones and twos" in society. We need to take something heterogeneous and treat it as though it were homogeneous. This is hard. Every nation struggles with this harsh reality. And to be fair, no single nation has gotten it right. The outside view, however, is that America struggles more deeply than others. Perhaps it is due to partisan politics and political myopia. Or perhaps Americans are happy with the system they have, which may or may not matter in the grand scheme of things since health and happiness are complicated bedfellows.

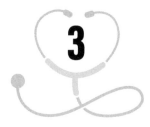

The UnHappiness Project

Happiness is the highest form of health.

—DALAI LAMA

Happiness, or subjective well-being as some refer to it, has long been associated with beneficial health outcomes at a population level. We can quibble and argue about the nuanced definitions of *happy* and *healthy* and how each of these variables should be measured, and I'll make the case that perhaps this is the crux of the problem: we can't seem to reasonably agree on broad or narrow definitions of either health or happiness in a consistent fashion. But for now, let's just accept at face value that a multitude of studies have shown a relationship between subjective well-being and some measure of improvement in overall health. Literature reviews and meta-analyses on happiness and health have generally concluded that happiness, or subjective well-being, can be beneficial to health.[1] Good health, however, is often recognized as the prerequisite to achieve happiness and well-being.[2] Research shows that happier people have been reported to be healthier people although it is difficult to assign causality to this relationship (more on that later).

But, then, why is everyone in health care so miserable? And does this misery translate into a meaningful impact on health? Life expectancy has increased in America for decades (save for a recent dip due to the opioid crisis). So, we're living longer, on average. But we're all miserable as far as health care is concerned. But happiness is associated with health. Huh?

Here is a nonempirical viewpoint, based on interactions and conversations with thousands of stakeholders in health care across more than two decades: Patients are unhappy with the whole thing—prices, access, quality of care, insurance. You name it. I cannot recall a single chronic patient that I have ever met who has raved about the health system and how efficiently it operates. And I'm not just saying that for dramatic effect. I mean, I really cannot cite a single example. I'm betting you can't either. Are many people happy that their disease is controlled or, better yet, cured? Of course. Are some people satisfied with their outcomes? No doubt. But is this happiness? Occasionally, you'll hear about a patient who went through an acute scenario and was pleasantly surprised at how it turned out. He presented at the local emergency department. It was not teeming with people. He was triaged quickly and effectively and seen by a physician within the first hour. Care was provided appropriately. Things that were happening to him were explained. He was discharged and no egregious bill followed six months later. Incidents like this are treated the same way we treat a UFO sighting or when someone swears they saw the Loch Ness Monster—we memorialize the event. And let's not confuse a patient who is grateful to their care team for, say, saving their life during an operation or delivering a healthy baby with what we're talking about here. Momentary gratitude is not remotely close to a deep, long-lasting sense of contentment with the system at large. Driven to emptying their bank accounts and near bankruptcy and beaten into submission by a system that doesn't speak their language, patients are resigned to the fact that the entire health care system's tagline could be summed up as "we're not happy, until you're not happy."

Let's not forget caregivers. They, too, are exhausted and equally disconsolate with the never-ending red tape of insurance paperwork and lengthy wait times as they shuttle their loved ones to and from appointments. This group of people is often overlooked in more than one way because we convince ourselves that caregiving doesn't really begin until one's later years. Not true. Caregiving is indiscriminate. At a younger age, you deal with sick parents or grandparents, and you have neither the experience nor the money to cope with the demands of the system. In your middle-aged years, you are sandwiched between raising a young family and trying to look after aging parents and relatives. And, in your own older years, you are busy worrying about your own health and, likely, worrying about the additional physical and emotional burden of looking after an equally old spouse or sibling. Happy? Far from it.

Doctors are burned out and despondent with a system that is nothing like what they imagined when they enrolled in medical school. It's the paperwork. It's the constant fighting against a system that doesn't seem to put the patient first. It's working conditions. It's compensation. Ditto for nurses and pharmacists. Politicians, too, are exasperated with spiraling costs and voter backlash at every turn. When their plan to raise enough money to pay for their grandiose health care vision is presented, they have to deal with political infighting and gridlock. Insurance companies and pharmacy benefits managers are crestfallen at the venom directed their way as they are blamed for the egregious costs imposed on the system. Patient advocacy groups, while doing incredibly important work, often struggle for funding and to find a clear voice that resonates and can move the needle on meaningful policy change on behalf of their membership. Manufacturers—both medical device and pharmaceutical—are no less miserable as they face a barrage of questions from lawmakers about their costs and pricing practices and a slew of disapproving looks from the general public about their perceived greed and callous approach to patients' lives. In fact, a recent Gallup Poll shows that the pharmaceutical industry is now the most poorly regarded industry in Americans' eyes, ranking last on a list of twenty-five industries.[3]

I know exactly what you're thinking. Healthy people are happy. They don't have to deal with cranky doctors, predatory insurance companies, expensive medicines, and burdening loved ones with their care needs. According to the Global Burden of Disease study of 2013 published in the *Lancet*, fewer than one in twenty people worldwide had no disease.[4] Correct. One in twenty. In other words, just 4.3 percent had no health problems while one-third of the earth's population reported more than five comorbidities. To bring this to a more identifiable level, think of twenty people you know. Nineteen of them have some sort of disease or illness. So, the obvious point is that there simply aren't that many healthy people around. And if you happen to be part of that lucky 4.3 percent, you're still not happy because you're grumbling about the fact that your tax dollars support social programs for which you get no value.

In 2018, See and Yen published a paper showing that happier nations have better health system performance as measured by efficiency.[5] They used the happiness index, which is a comprehensive indicator that includes several important components, such as, caring, freedom, generosity, honesty, health, income, and good governance. They measured efficiency as a function of life expectancy and inverse mortality rates. The findings show that happiness is one of the factors that contributes to the efficiency of a country's health system. Others have also published similar results on the topic of happiness and health. But health system efficiency is not the holy grail. We're not after the relationship between happiness and health system efficiency. We're interested in the relationship between happiness and actual health. Or are we? Maybe health system efficiency is a good surrogate marker since measures of health are up for endless debate. Do we use life expectancy? Or infant mortality rates? Maybe we should use hospital readmission rates or maternal mortality? So, it seems, definitions are important.

Here's another way of looking at it. Let's take the results from the General Social Survey. The GSS gathers data on contemporary American society in order to monitor and explain trends and constants in attitudes, behaviors, and attributes. Hundreds of trends have been tracked since 1972. It is the only full-probability, personal-interview survey designed to monitor changes in both social characteristics and attitudes currently conducted in the United States, and it is managed by the National Opinion Research Center at the University of Chicago.[6] Let's look at the relationship between health and happiness using actual questions to actual humans (not life expectancy data and inverse mortality rates).

The chart of GSS data is fascinating for a variety of reasons (figure 6). Let's unpack them. First, it reinforces what we intuitively know to be true: there is a large gap in happiness between those who self-report being in excellent health compared to being in poor health. In the most recent year of data collection (2018), the GSS shows that only 11 percent of people in poor health rate themselves as "very happy," whereas 52 percent of respondents in excellent health rate themselves the same way. Another interesting observation is the surprising drop off in happiness from "excellent" health to "good" health. The graph depicts an almost halving in self-reported happiness from 52 percent to 27 percent when respondents declare their health as excellent versus good. The obvious interpretation is that health is a critical component of individual happiness, demonstrated by the fact that even the smallest (one level) move in health has a tremendous effect on happiness. Or, it could indicate

Response: Very happy
Breakdown: Condition of health

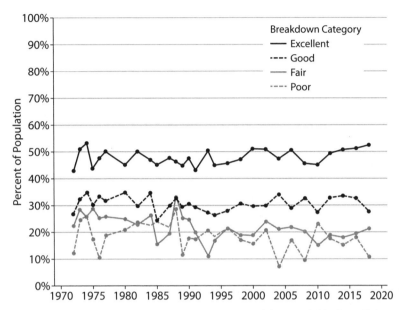

Figure 6. General Social Surveys, 1972–2018 (machine-readable data file). Tom W. Smith, Michael Davern, Jeremy Freese, and Stephen Morgan, sponsored by National Science Foundation (Chicago: National Opinion Research Council, 2018; NORC at the University of Chicago [producer and distributor]). Data accessed from the GSS Data Explorer, gssdataexplorer.norc.org.

that, depending on when you surveyed people, individuals have not fully adapted to a recent health change, and this lack of adaptation manifests as low happiness scores. In other words, if you sampled the same people twelve months later, the gap might not be so large because they would have adapted to their new health state (see more on this subject below). About a decade ago (2010), the GSS results showed that people in the worst health state (poor health) self-declared as happier than people in fair health. And, in fact, in this same year, the "poor" health group had almost the same level of "very happy" as the "good" health group (23% vs. 27%).

Now, take a look at figure 7. What do you make of it? This is the same data set, but instead of looking at those who are "very

Response: Very happy
Breakdown: Condition of health

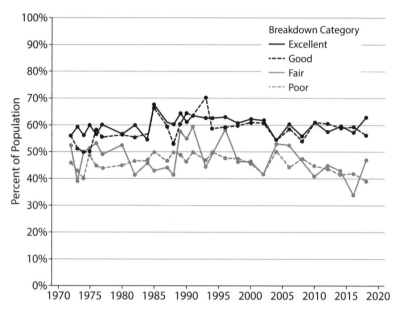

Figure 7. General Social Surveys, 1972–2018 (machine-readable data file). Tom W. Smith, Michael Davern, Jeremy Freese, and Stephen Morgan. Sponsored by National Science Foundation (Chicago: National Opinion Research Council, 2018; NORC at the University of Chicago [producer and distributor]). Data accessed from the GSS Data Explorer, gssdataexplorer.norc.org.

happy," we are looking at people who declare themselves to be "pretty happy." Do you notice the clustering of the data points between the 40 percent and 60 percent level? Basically, the happiness band is tighter. What this tells us (soberingly) is that to just be "pretty happy," your health status may not be as important as it is for being "very happy." Maybe other determinants play a larger role in what I'll call basic happiness, such as income, education, and interpersonal relationships. Maybe the association between health and happiness is most explicit and pronounced at the highest levels of happiness. Maybe there is a happiness hierarchy that relies on lower-order elements to get us to basic happiness and higher-order elements that take us to advanced happiness. Or maybe this tells us that, when we rely on self-reported levels of happiness and health, there is bound to be some "noise."

Perhaps one of the most important voices in happiness research belongs to Richard Easterlin (he's so famous he has a paradox named after him, the Easterlin Paradox). His seminal work has focused on happiness and income growth, but he does address happiness and health.[7] And while he doesn't propose a unifying solution to the problem of the relationship between health and happiness, Easterlin goes out of his way to address the prevailing viewpoint that there is some sort of adaptation to declining health and that this adaptation impacts happiness. By sharing the conclusions of a few landmark studies,

> these results suggest that, on average, an adverse change in health reduces life satisfaction, and the worse the change in health, the greater the reduction in life satisfaction. The results do not mean that no adaptation to disability occurs. The initial impact on happiness, say, of an accident or serious disease, is no doubt greater than its long-term impact. Adjustment to a disabling condition may be facilitated by health devices such as hearing aids, medications, or wheelchairs, and by a support network of friends and relatives. Moreover, the extent of adaptation may vary depending on the personality or other characteristics of the individual affected. But the evidence does suggest that, even with adaptation, there is, on average, a lasting negative effect on happiness of an adverse change in health.[8]

And then there's the United Nations *World Happiness Report 2017*, which shows that among the top twenty happiest nations on the planet, a healthy life expectancy matters in the overall happiness equation but accounts for less of a nation's overall happiness than, perhaps, we think (figure 8). This doesn't necessarily contradict any of the peer-reviewed work out there as the empirical data are very clear that health is only *one* of the myriad factors associated with happiness. But what the UN *World Happiness Report* reinforces is that the impact of health might be even less than we think. It might also suggest that a healthy life expectancy is quite honestly an awkward way to assess the relationship between health and happiness. Once again, we are forced to grapple with the reality that the definition of these variables may be the issue. The time series of healthy life expectancy at birth are constructed based on data from the World Health Organization and Word Development Indicators. First, the authors generate the ratios of healthy life expectancy to life expectancy in 2012 for countries with both data. They then apply the country-specific ratios to other years to generate the healthy life expectancy data.[9] In short, no one was asked a simple question like, *How much of your happiness is related to your current health status?* And perhaps for good reason since the responses might have been difficult to interpret. Having said that, the same report uses open-ended questions about corruption, generosity, and freedom to determine levels for

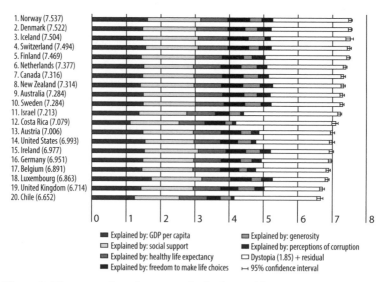

Figure 8. The twenty happiest countries in the world. J. Helliwell, R. Layard, and J. Sachs, *World Happiness Report 2017* (New York: Sustainable Development Solutions Network, 2017).

these variables. The point I'm trying to make is that these questions are as difficult to ask as they are to answer.

To further muddy the waters, the World Health Organization defines health as "a state of complete physical, mental and social well being and not merely the absence of disease or infirmity."[10] In a letter to the *British Medical Journal* in 1997, Rodolfo Saracci, the director of research in epidemiology at the National Research Council in Pisa, Italy, makes the observation that "a state of complete physical, mental, and social wellbeing corresponds much more closely to happiness than to health."[11] So there's that. The consequence of getting the definition of health and happiness all topsy-turvy, according to Saracci, is that we are trying to attain the unattainable—happiness for everybody. And in doing so, we are misallocating resources and effort that could be directed at the "gradually attainable"—which is health equity for all. But it is another point he makes about this tortuous health-happiness balancing act that we seem obsessed with that is far more germane. Saracci claims that since the quest for happiness is never-ending the quest for health becomes never-ending, too. By virtue of the inability or unwillingness to decouple these two concepts, we legitimize the pursuit of everlasting health. And, in doing so, perhaps we send an inadvertent message that provides tacit permission to people to use more resources.

The upshot of all this? As with everything health care related, this is a complicated topic. There are methodological issues with all these articles, opinion surveys, and reports. How do we measure happiness? How do we measure health? And health system efficiency? Is there a link between the two? Do efficient health systems produce healthier patients? Is there another variable that is a better surrogate marker for health than health system efficiency? Is there an inherent selection bias in our data? Or other biases that we are not aware of? And, of course, how do we define these variables? I mean, it's all confusing, isn't it? If happiness is important at both an individual level and a societal level in contributing to health, why are so many people so unhappy with the state of health care. If so many people are unhappy with the state of health care, how is it that we are producing this efficiency in certain countries? Maybe the answer is that other variables related to happiness (such as income, education, housing, good government, security, religious freedom, etc.) mask or overwhelm the low numbers associated with happiness from health care. Or, as the UN *World Happiness Report* shows, maybe the extent to which health accounts for happiness is actually less than we think. Maybe the simple answer is that people aren't as happy as we think they are. Regardless, this much is true: health and happiness are associated. This is a fact that has been presented in the peer-reviewed literature for decades and a topic on which volumes of work have been based without question as to its validity or veracity. But it's a messy relationship. There is confusion over which direction the causality flows. Perhaps the most important takeaway from all of this is that even if we knew the answers to all these questions, would we be any happier or healthier?

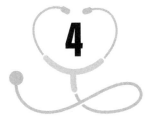

Customer Satisfaction

There are two ways to get enough. One is to continue to accumulate more and more. The other is to desire less.

—G. K. CHESTERTON

It's happening everywhere in nations in the Organisation for Economic Co-operation and Development and even in emerging health markets. And if it's not happening in your jurisdiction, it's sure to happen soon. The *it* is tying a portion of health care funding to patient satisfaction.

The problems with this new movement are obvious and lengthy. What are we measuring? Is it defined the same way by patients everywhere? Is there a standardized perspective for calculating and grading patient satisfaction? Are providers and patients both on the same page with respect to patient satisfaction goals?

In Europe and North America, we are talking big numbers. Nearly $1 billion in payments to hospitals in the United States alone over the next few years will be based in part on patient satisfaction, determined by a twenty-seven-question government survey administered to patients. Hospitals with high scores will get a bonus payment. Those with low ones will lose money.[1] In the United Kingdom up to 10 percent of the payments to National Health Service trusts are dependent on adequate levels of patient satisfaction.[2] In Canada, the government of Ontario, the most populous province, has instituted a mandatory patient satisfaction survey and patient complaints process as part of the new funding mechanism.[3] And the list goes on.

Survey questions in the United States included, "How often did doctors treat you with courtesy and respect?" "How often were your room and bathroom kept clean?" It asked patients to rate their stay on a scale of 0 to 10. A senior nurse at a 953-bed facility in the United States, cited a patient who had a hemorrhagic stroke and recovered swiftly enough to walk out of the hospital about a week later. On the survey, the patient complained that meals were served cold and gave the hospital low scores.[4] In Canada, survey questions included, "After you knew that you needed to be admitted to a hospital bed, did you have to wait too long before getting there?" "When you left the hospital, did you have a better understanding of your condition than when you entered?" "Before giving you any new medicine, how often did hospital staff describe possible side effects in a way you could understand?"[5]

This smattering of questions illustrates an important point: Are we interested in better outcomes, increasing health literacy, hotel factors, or some combination of all three? The temperature of the food, the cleanliness of the rooms, the proximity to elevators and hospital parking spaces are all part of the patient experience. No argument. To what extent do these hotel factors contribute to better outcomes? They don't. Providers know that and so do patients. To use two stark examples to drive home the point: Lowering the parking fees at your hospital won't shrink your tumor. The increased punctuality of your meal delivery won't alleviate the excruciating pain associated with your severe rheumatoid arthritis.

We need to consider other important aspects of patient satisfaction, such as the difference across these factors in an acute care versus a chronic care facility or the difference in satisfaction scores between primary care and specialty care. What expectations do patients have anyway? Do first-time hospital visitors rate hospitals higher because they have no measuring stick against which to gauge? Are patients even qualified to be able to distinguish between high-value and low-value health care? Do they even know what it looks like, or more precisely, do they even know what to look for? How many ratings are absent and free of the influence of the caregiver (a child visits his or her elderly parent in the hospital and is appalled at the treatment and fills out the satisfaction survey for the parent not knowing half of what goes on)? Perhaps one of the biggest questions of them all when it comes to patient satisfaction is, Are we really measuring satisfaction, or are we (loosely) measuring some form of happiness?

We've all heard the arguments for this system: we need to hold providers and hospital systems accountable. The private sector (banks, airlines, fast-food chains, etc.) is obsessive about customer satisfaction—why shouldn't the public sector be the same way? I agree. We do need to hold providers and hospitals accountable, and we do need some degree of the "voice of the customer" as part of the solution in this accountability push. But this way is not working in my view. Yes, the private sector has some great ideas. Actually, we don't need to look at banks and airlines for answers. There is private health care. There are procedures and treatments offered outside the public system. The plastic surgeries, the dermatology centers (Botox), the laser-vision correction centers are all excellent analogs for policy makers to examine for a real-world litmus test of patient satisfaction. The threshold is presumably much higher because no private or public payer is footing the bill. In other words, these patients are a really tough audience to please because they pay out of their own pockets.

MISUNDERSTANDING HEALTH 40

Trying to unpack this argument or issue is no easy task. But let's try. On the issue of whether we're measuring the same thing or whether there is a standardized approach to measuring patient satisfaction, the answer is a resounding no. We're not there yet. Herein lies the problem. When you tie funding to patient satisfaction scores and you're using different systems (all of which are unvalidated), there are bound to be some winners and some losers. More precisely, there are bound to be some winners who shouldn't be winners and losers who shouldn't be losers. Some hospitals and health systems are bound to get screwed. And when one hospital gets less in funding because their patient satisfaction scores are lower than the median or some predetermined target, guess what happens? Services get cut. Care is rationed. Oh, and believe it or not, some hospitals and health systems will game the system to try and improve their scores to get that funding back in the next fiscal year. John Sitzia's research out of the United Kingdom from 1999, which looked at the validity and reliability of patient satisfaction data from 195 studies, clearly supports the notion that a lack of standardization plagues the field of patient satisfaction research.[6] Sitzia states that "a large majority of published investigations of patient satisfaction use instruments which are untested or barely tested. It must be concluded that the results from such studies lack credibility." Until we all start asking the right questions and collecting the answers the same way, we have a problem. It's not some existential question debated over cigars and brandy snifters by policy wonks. It's a pragmatic problem that requires our attention: Why are we tying important and badly needed funding dollars to unvalidated, untested, and nonstandardized instruments? The solution is not to decouple patient satisfaction measures from funding but to develop a standard survey or test that can be used across multiple settings and that has wide generalizability.

Let's assume we get that part right. Here's the other problem. Even if we ask the right questions and collect answers the right way, we need to find some meaningful way to link patient satisfaction to health outcomes. Don't we? Is it any good to have a health system that has a bunch of customers who are satisfied with everything except the one thing we're most interested in impacting, which is their overall health? Let's assume that people who are sick understand that the taste of their food, the cost of the hospital parking, and the way their doctor speaks to them really has no effect on their disease and/or their ability to get better. It's a safe assumption. No? Then why are we interested in patient satisfaction? If it has no impact on outcomes and even patients know it has no impact on outcomes, does any of this matter?

Well, it turns out that it might matter, provided we look beyond the hotel factors. Boulding et al. looked at the thirty-day readmission rates in a sample of 1,798 hospitals for acute myocardial infarction, 2,561 hospitals for heart failure, and 2,562 hospitals for pneumonia and correlated those rates with patient satisfaction scores. What the researchers found was that higher overall patient satisfaction scores were associated with lower thirty-day risk-standardized readmission rates for all three clinical conditions at a highly statistically significant level ($P < .001$).[7] This, with limited generalizability and recognition of the fact that the data are cross-sectional in nature, which precludes any causal inference, provides some good preliminary evidence that, indeed, we can link patient satisfaction to tangible and meaningful health outcome measures. For further ammunition, see table 2. It presents the argument that patient satisfaction is "less about trying to make patients 'happy' (e.g., improving the food or the decor of the room) and the hotel factors that I have been referring to and is more about increasing the quality of their interactions with hospital personnel, especially nurses and physicians," as evidenced by the fact that, aside from pain management, four of the top five dimensions of self-reported patient satisfaction in the Boulding et al. study are related to communication and provider-patient interactions in some way.[8]

Table 2. Pairwise correlations of HCAHPS-reported dimensions
of quality and overall patient satisfaction

Variable	Correlation Coefficient
How often did nurses communicate well with patients?	0.845
How often was patient's pain well controlled?	0.805
How often did patients receive help quickly from hospital staff?	0.776
How often did staff explain about medicines before giving them to patients?	0.740
How often did doctors communicate well with patients?	0.695
How often were the patients' rooms and bathrooms kept clean?	0.675
Patient satisfaction with discharge planning	0.638
How often was the area around patients' rooms kept quiet at night?	0.611

Note: HCAHPS = Hospital Consumer Assessment of Healthcare Providers and Systems.

The other reason that all this matters is that the subtler aspects of patient satisfaction measures may indeed play a larger role in healing even though this role is not well understood. Compassion, respect, empathy, feeling connected, and being heard are important elements of recovery and healing. Manary et al. published an interesting paper elucidating aspects of this topic.[9] The premise of their paper and their research was that patient satisfaction might foretell the quality of care provided. What they found, among other things, was that when patient satisfaction is measured as a function of a single, distinct visit, there is a strong correlation with satisfaction scores and outcomes, such as mortality and readmission rates. This is exactly what we want. We want the dollars that we are allocating to patient satisfaction measures to show that a patient's satisfaction actually means something in the long run. It should come as no surprise that the timeliness of the patient satisfaction survey is critically important in establishing the relationship as well. Some of the better instruments such as the HCAHPS (Hospital Consumer Assessment of Healthcare Providers and Systems) collect data no later than forty-two days after the patient's discharge, whereas a typical survey deployed by a health plan may ask patients to recall experiences that occurred over a year ago, which can introduce recall biases.[10]

We know that not all survey instruments are created equal. We know that we've got to be a little more disciplined about when we deploy surveys and that we need to ensure that patient satisfaction is measured, ideally, against a single visit as opposed to some vague time frame that stretches across months or even years. Fine. But what about cost? Do satisfied patients cost the system less money?

Fenton et al. looked at the relationship between patient satisfaction and health care utilization, expenditures, and mortality in a nationally representative sample and published their results a few years ago.[11] Here's how it worked: Anyone aged eighteen and over who reported at least one clinic/physician visit in the previous year was included in the study. Respondents were then asked about their satisfaction levels pertaining to that visit. Their patient satisfaction score was measured according to four items linked to physician communication; specifically, how often in the past twelve months the physician or other health care provider performed these four tasks (table 3).

A fifth item in which patients rated their health care from all physicians and other health care providers on a scale of 0 to 10 (from the worst to the best health care possible) was also incorporated. These five items comprised the satisfaction score in year 1 based on some previous visit in what we'll call year 0. Then, the

Table 3. Patient satisfaction scores measured according to four items linked to physician communication

1. Listened carefully
2. Explained things in a way that was easy to understand
3. Showed respect for what they had to say
4. Spent enough time with them

same people were followed to track health care utilization and expenditure in year 2. So, in a nutshell, let's say that someone you know had a health care visit or an interaction today. And then sometime in the next year, you asked her about her satisfaction with that visit. And then for a year after that, you tracked her health care utilization and expenditure. This would be how the Fenton et al. study was set up.

Surprisingly, the most satisfied patients cost the system the most money (compared to the least satisfied patients) as far as total health care expenditure and prescription drug expenditure are concerned. Remember the design of this study: satisfaction in year 1 was correlated with expenditure in year 2—and *only* year 2. In other words, if this study had followed drug and total health care expenditures for a longer time frame, it is quite conceivable that drug and total health care expenditures might have evened out or not been significantly different between the most and least satisfied groups. A potential explanation for this strange result is that satisfaction was largely measured as a function of physician communication. It's possible that the most satisfied patients are the ones who find their physicians provided them with validation for interventions and treatments that drove resource utilization. That is, if I tell my doctor that I'm depressed and that I'd like to try a course of antidepressant treatment along with a referral to a psychiatrist and he agrees with me, I am likely to rate him highly on a communication-satisfaction survey because he "showed respect for what I had to say" and "listened carefully" to my viewpoint (table 3). In this scenario, I'm also going to be getting a prescription drug and a referral to a psychiatrist—both of which will drive cost in the "most satisfied" category to which I belong. Conversely, if I have the same conversation with another doctor who doesn't "communicate as well" and "doesn't listen to me," he might determine that it's premature for a prescription and a referral. I would then rate him lower on the satisfaction scale, and, naturally, my total health care and drug expenditure costs would be lower compared to someone who was more satisfied because I never got the drug or the referral. We need to be cautious about our interpretation of these data, and much more work is needed. The argument is not that physicians ought to listen less or show less respect for their patients but that patient satisfaction may be a function of variables outside of the traditional health care system and, at the very least, mediated by far more than simply having a good communication relationship with a provider. It's complicated.

But I am being deliberate about explaining all these various study designs and interpreting the results for you because this topic of patient satisfaction has important implications. Some will argue that if we're going to ask the wrong people the wrong questions, perhaps we need not even ask the questions at all. My argument is this: at the end of the day, people are paying for services—whether through payroll deductions, the public purse, out-of-pocket costs, or private health insurance premiums—and people ought to be satisfied with services rendered for which they are required to pay. Yes, it's true that we are struggling with instrument validation, grappling with the actual definition of "satisfaction," and recognizing that we need to decide between assessing hotel factors and communication elements of the patient-provider relationship, which, it seems, are a more meaningful measure of patient satisfaction. Whether this patient satisfaction need translates into something meaningful through lower costs or better outcomes to justify the policy effort and the handwringing is truly open to debate. It may turn out that we are happy with high satisfaction scores simply on their own. We need to recognize that, if we can't crack this nut—if we continue to misunderstand the drivers of satisfaction—patients are going to start looking for their own answers and drawing their own conclusions.

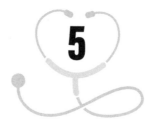

5

I Still Haven't Found What I'm Looking For

Seeking what is true is not seeking what is desirable.
—ALBERT CAMUS, *The Myth of Sisyphus and Other Essays*

Recently, my neighbor Maria shared a story with me about her experience with "Dr. Google." She'd discovered a red splotch on her left forearm. She didn't know where it had come from but decided to dismiss it. It didn't hurt. A day later the discoloration was worse, and there was some itching and some pain. She wore a long sleeve shirt to cover it up. On day three, however, the pain intensified. She knew she needed to take some action. So, she started googling symptoms and diagnoses for "red skin discoloration" and other permutations of that phrase. She found some images. And some advice. And she also found some ads for creams and lotions.

Approximately 4.5 percent of all internet searches are for health-related information. In the United States alone, six million people search for health-related information each day, which exceeds the combined number of daily outpatient visits to emergency departments and physician offices.[1] In all, 80 percent of internet users, or about 93 million Americans, have searched for a health-related topic online, according to a study released by the Pew Research Center's Internet & American Life Project in July 2019. That's up from 62 percent of internet users who said they went online to research health topics in 2001, the Washington research firm found. The Pew researchers asked participants whether they had used the internet to search for at least one of sixteen major health topics online, ranging from mental health and immunizations to sexual health information. Most frequently, people went online to look up information about a specific disease or medical problem (63%) or a particular medical treatment or procedure (47%). They were also interested in diet, nutrition, and vitamins (44%) and exercise or fitness information (36%).[2] This group has been coined *health seekers* and most of them go online at least once a month for health information.

Peer-reviewed literature has attempted to better understand the profile of people who use search engines for access to health information. A fair number of papers have attempted to answer how patients perceive the quality of this information, the degree to which patients share the information they find with their clinician, and the seasonal trends associated with health information seeking. But, in truth, we should start with a very simple question: What are health seekers fundamentally looking for? In other words, can we reveal patient priorities using search engines in relation to health seeking to make meaningful policy changes that affect the way health information is contextualized and retrieved.

The literature, along with richly detailed reports from organizations such as the Pew Research Center and the Commonwealth Fund, shows that most health seekers use online search engines as a starting point to gain information on a disease or illness or to seek information on the treatment options for a particular disease or illness. While health seekers also look to better understand costs, to find information about potential providers, and to understand support group resources, there is no ambiguity that health seekers are essentially looking for information about their disease and how to treat it. To no one's surprise, Google is by far the most popular search engine in the United States and accounts for over 85 percent of health-related searches. We also know that almost four out of five health seekers (77%) start an online health information search by accessing Google, Bing, and Yahoo! with just 13 percent saying that they begin at a site that specializes in health information (such as WebMD), and less than 2 percent of health seekers will start at a social media platform such as Wikipedia or Facebook.[3] This is very intuitive and completely unsurprising, but perhaps what is surprising is that these results hold true across a variety of diseases, from laser vision correction to oncology to back pain and that there appears to be no difference according to age or gender. However, the timing of health information seeking does appear to exhibit some differences in revealing health-seeking priorities: health seekers looking for information for themselves tend to do so before seeing a clinician, whereas those looking on behalf of someone tend to seek information after a visit with a doctor.

While our gut instinct is to roll our eyes at this type of behavior, let's be clear that online health information seeking can benefit us. It can, for instance, potentially increase health literacy and can also lead to greater engagement in disease management, which in turn may be associated with better compliance and better outcomes. It also helps counteract the lingering effects of an overly paternalistic approach to health care, back when many doctors were apt to give their patients a figurative pat on the head. *There, there now. Let the doctor make all the decisions for you.* You may remember a time when the principal-agent relationship as described in health care was the dominant strategy. In this scenario, the doctor acted as the agent and the patient as the principal, and their ensuing relationship was governed to a large extent by the deferral of that patient's property rights. In other words, when the orthopedic surgeon told

Mrs. Smith that she had a degenerative hip condition and needed hip replacement surgery and that she could choose between the titanium hip, the steel hip, or the cobalt-chromium hip, Mrs. Smith would naturally defer her property rights and ask the surgeon, "I'll take whatever you think is best for me."

But that model is largely gone. Using search engines to get more information about our health upends the traditional doctor-patient relationship. It's not all bad. Rather, health-seeking behavior has given rise to a shared decision-making model in contrast to the principal-agent relationship. This shared decision-making model, ideally, is one in which doctors and patients work together to achieve disease management that fits patients' needs. Studies have supported the notion that the use of online health information seeking may be beneficial. Van Riel et al. reported the results of over seven hundred patients involved in an observational, cross-sectional study that looked at the role of online health information–seeking behavior prior to seeing a primary care physician and the resulting impact on actions and behaviors of the study sample.[4] It may be fairly obvious to the keen reader that the study design here (observational and cross-sectional) is not the most robust, because confounding is a natural problem with observational data sets and cross-sectional data are marked by an approach in which the exposure and the outcome are determined at the same point in time in a given population. Therefore, it is difficult to establish causal inference, and the temporal relationship between the exposure and the outcome cannot normally be determined. For example, if drinking milk is associated with peptic ulcer, is that because milk causes ulcers or because persons with ulcers drink milk to relieve their symptoms? Nonetheless, this type of study is informative in its own way. And what Van Riel et al. show us is that most health seekers in their study are women under the age of sixty, and over 75 percent go to the general practitioner at least once a year. The study also elucidates that responders who frequently visited the GP more often went to a consultation after their search on the internet ($P<.0001$). Patients who frequently consult their doctor more often presented with an increase in anxiety ($P<.0001$) and noticed additional complaints after the online search ($P=.0065$). Both eye-opening associations strain existing and finite resources and result in an increased level of sequelae, which may or may not be associated with diagnosed disease.

Interestingly, the authors report that responders who frequently searched online health information often decided not to go to the doctor ($P<.0001$) and took medication more often without the advice of the GP ($P=.0011$). Of course, these are some of the challenges in this new system, many of which will be familiar to those who have consulted Dr. Google: possible delayed diagnosis, convincing yourself you don't have something when you really do, wasted trips to the doctor, trying your own home remedy (a.k.a. taking medications without the advice of a doctor), and so on. Yet, in all these potential pitfalls, we rarely consider a more troubling question: What role does Google itself play in all this?

As outlined previously, most health seekers use online search engines as a starting point to gain information on a disease or to seek information on the treatment options for a particular disease; Google is their most popular search engine by far. But, in 2017 Google was fined an incredible $2.4 billion in the European Union for skewing its search results;[5] therefore, it's worth considering the corresponding implications for online health information seeking. According to the EU regulator's investigation into Google's practices, the company's search algorithm systematically and consistently gave prominent placement to its own services, to the detriment of rival services. This skew is critical to the health care context, as the ten highest-ranking generic search results on page one receive approximately 95 percent of all clicks. In a health care search scenario, this means that when my neighbor Maria looks up her symptoms, the search results might potentially show information on an "amazing" cream or ointment. Those results could be entirely based on the advertising dollars a company has spent, as well as on the corresponding search engine optimization used to vault it to page one.

It doesn't help that health seekers are, by and large, incapable of distinguishing between high-value (i.e., correct) and low-value (i.e., incorrect) health care information. If you take people who can't reasonably tell what is accurate and what is not, and you introduce content on the first page of a search result, it would not be surprising for those individuals to assume that what comes first must be the most important. This is a rather mundane behavioral insight, which has huge implications when it comes to how we certify, adjudicate, and validate online health information—an entirely different topic on its own but worth mentioning because of the obvious link to the whole subject of online health information seeking. Why do we even care about all this? We care because there are approximately seventy thousand websites/online platforms that purport to provide health information. They can't all be saying the same thing, and they can't all be right. Additional sources show that approximately 70 percent of studies that assess the quality of online platforms' ability and accuracy in delivering health information, report grossly inaccurate or misleading information on a significant proportion of these portals.[6] Because a significant proportion of these gateways to health information may be inaccurate in their information, this has the potential to drive unexpected cost to the system.

Daraz et al. published a systematic review on the overall quality of online health information.[7] The authors looked at "3393 references and included 153 cross-sectional studies evaluating 11,785 websites using 14 quality assessment tools. The quality level varied across scales. Using DISCERN, none of the websites received a category of excellent in quality, 37–79% were rated as good, and the rest were rated as poor quality." This is crucial because DISCERN is an instrument designed to provide users with a reliable way to measure the quality of written health information. It was originally developed by Deborah Charnock, Sasha Shepperd, Gill Needham, and Robert Gann, who reported on its development and validation in a February 1999 paper.[8] DISCERN is designed for use by individual consumers, health information providers, and health professionals, and the instrument contains fifteen questions that may be rated on a scale of 1 to 5 with questions intended to draw user attention to issues of potential bias, content currency, relevance, clarity, evidence, and balance.

Thus, the importance of understanding what health seekers are looking for has important implications for policy makers in that it can help guide decisions through the allocation of resources to underserved or needy segments of the population and eradicate misinformation and inefficiency associated with self-diagnosis, which may lead to regulation or certification of the way in which online health information is made available. That is, while searching the web for health information can bring benefit, it can also bring harm. Instead of writing it off entirely, I'd argue that what we really need is regulation and oversight. This is a bold approach for an industry and for a policy issue already drowning in regulation. Health information is not the same as celebrity gossip, but it is information; it should be available and reliable. So far, no tangible solutions have emerged, despite best efforts. One obvious reason is that it's hard to govern information on the web where anyone with a credit card and a GoDaddy account can set up shop.

We also don't have good quality signals to send to consumers who are looking for health information. This may be an easier fix: if we assigned a top-level domain, such as ".health," people could use it as a signal that a website has been reviewed and adjudicated for accuracy and completeness. Until then, everyone is left to their own interpretation. Although it's sometimes easy to tell when a web page is from a reputable clinical source (i.e., Mayo Clinic), other times it isn't. Then there's the issue of consensus. Suppose there was some person or group regulating online health information. Where would that person or group gain consensus on what information should be shared online? In medicine, the heterogeneity of disease combined with a patient's own underlying comorbidities makes it nearly impossible to suggest a specific treatment approach for every single patient or to provide a boilerplate solution to a majority of disease scenarios. Aside from basic scientific information and definitions, the lack of consensus is a real barrier.

It is complicated.

We want people engaged in their health care. We want higher levels of health literacy (defined as "the degree to which individuals have the capacity to obtain, process and understand basic health information and services needed to make appropriate health decisions"[9]). We want patients learning about their disease and their treatment options so that they can increase their odds of successful outcomes—because research shows that people who are better informed about their health status are more likely to have better outcomes. Let me be more precise: differences in health literacy levels have been consistently associated with increased hospitalizations, greater emergency care use, lower use of mammography, lower receipt of influenza vaccine, poorer ability to demonstrate taking medications appropriately, poorer ability to interpret labels and health messages, and, among elderly people, poorer overall health status and higher mortality.[10]

The downsides of online health information–seeking behavior are real and tangible: Fake information. Sophisticated search engine optimization tools designed to skew content. Low health literacy.

What is abundantly clear is that people aren't about to stop using Dr. Google. If we ignore the downsides, things will get worse, as they usually do. Individuals will continue to make decisions about their own health care, even though they are grossly incapable of making such decisions. The unchecked growth of inaccurate, bogus sites could also nurture a nation of vigilant, search engine–using hypochondriacs. Or a nation of health information-seeking skeptics who no longer trust anything they read online even though it may be clinically important. Although already burdened with a tremendous amount of paperwork and with crushing amounts of clinical responsibility, a group of potential gatekeepers lie among us. Who else better than their current doctor, nurse practitioner, or pharmacist to better guide them in pursuit of accurate and meaningful online health information? This is the unfortunate problem about health care: it is built on informational asymmetry. By virtue of specialized training and experience, your doctor is (largely) the only one who can validate or reject the health information you find. He or she has an asymmetric amount and degree of information. It's not as though your dry cleaner can determine whether the online health information you found is accurate. Or your banker. Or your car mechanic.

Here's what I tell people: Think of this as a palindromic problem. It is the identical problem both frontward and backward. Without some sort of meaningful intervention, we might drive people to seek care when none is required, or we might drive them to avoid care when care is required. Either way, doing nothing is also a less-than-optimal outcome. The last thing we need in health care is another less-than-optimal outcome. At the end of the day, understanding what, how, and when patients typically seek information about health care and having a strictly enforced global system that puts limits on the ability of paid advertising to influence search query results in health information seeking is critical.

Otherwise, none of us may ever find what we're looking for. While some may advance the notion that not finding what we're looking for is just a part of life, there are some scenarios when it can be a both a blessing and a curse.

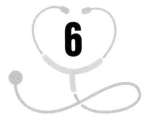

6

The Rating Game

> When you develop your opinions on the basis of weak evidence, you will have difficulty interpreting subsequent information that contradicts these opinions, even if this new information is obviously more accurate.
>
> —Nassim Nicholas Taleb, *The Black Swan: The Impact of the Highly Improbable*

Society's obsession with rating everything has real implications for health care. And those implications are not all good.

After the brutal American elections of both 2016 and 2020, it is clear that fake news may have played a role in shaping the opinions of millions and millions of voters before and after the outcome. Why is that important? Because there is a corollary to health care. Fake news is often disguised as opinion and can be a euphemism for *user generated content*. That is not to say that every opinion posted on the internet is intentionally fake or designed to mislead, but it may very well be interpreted as authentic simply by virtue of being published or posted online. You and I might know better. But not everyone does. When you are desperate (i.e., looking for a doctor or a treatment for a disease), you may be willing to overlook some of these inconveniences. Here's the upshot of what you're about to read: how do we validate, authenticate, and allow the posting of user generated content in a manner that still allows freedom of expression and thought but doesn't drive the underinformed to make decisions that are bad for their welfare? (I think I'm still talking about health care and not the election of an American president.)

Ask yourself this simple question: How would you like it if someone showed up at your job, spent seven to twelve minutes with you, and then posted an opinion of your competency on a widely viewed website? What if that person had an axe to grind or didn't really have the competency to understand whether you were good at your job? What if that person was not really rating you but was rating a colleague, such as a receptionist or a nurse who worked with you? What if you were just having an off day?

This is happening every day on sites such as CareDash, Yelp, Vitals, and RateMDs. And there is absolutely nothing wrong with expressing an opinion about the demeanor of the receptionist, the wait time, the décor of the office, the lack of parking, or the bed-side manner of a clinician. In fact, some of this feedback and in-put can be valuable. But when these online sites start accepting random reviews and comments about a clinician's professional competency (i.e., misdiagnosis of a condition or recommendation for a particular treatment approach that was later disputed by a second opinion) or allow allegations about supposed overbilling and innuendo of fraud, we've gone too far. Let's be clear: the suggestion is not that clinicians are above criticism but, rather, that the criticism be a fair reflection of the complainant's ability to provide meaningful insight. There is a vast difference between making a complaint based on behavior and a complaint based on competency. There's a vast difference between making a complaint to a governing body such as the American Medical Association, which has a clear mechanism for submitting a complaint about a physician—a relatively anonymous process—and posting a review online for all to see and for all to search.

I had the chance to speak with Ted Chan, the founder and CEO of CareDash, about the rationale and motivation behind sites like his that attempt to help patients improve their experience at finding a doctor that meets their needs. It started, he told me, with the frustrating search for health care information for a loved one. He found himself poring over hundreds of web pages of information with varying degrees of authenticity. So, like all curious and driven entrepreneurs, he thought he could do something about his problem and turn it into a business at the same time. When I spoke to him, CareDash had three hundred thousand unique reviews posted by patients based on interactions with a health care provider and approximately two million patients visiting the site per month. When I brought up the issue of sites like CareDash as being opinion sites, he acknowledged that his team is working on making data substantively more outcomes-based and objective, but he did concede that there would always be an element of opinion embedded in doctor reviews. There is no debate, as Chan points out, that consumers are looking for more transparency in health care. The question is whether transparency is achieved through the reviews of complete strangers who may or may not be skilled at interpreting and converting their interactions with health care providers into a meaningful insight for other consumers.

And here is why I say we need to be clear, why I think we have gone too far, and why this is important: tons of people are reading these reviews for more than just a good laugh. You're thinking exactly what I'm thinking: *Do people really scour these review sites looking for a doctor? Do people really make decisions on provider care based on the random comments (positive or negative) of complete strangers?* Yes, they do. Some unpublished estimates[1] suggest that upward of 25 percent of health seekers will find their doctor on-line while other more recent market research suggests the number might be somewhere between 60 percent and 75 percent when looking at consumers who take online reviews into account and are influenced by online feedback in their search for a doctor.[2] And this growing dependence on and trust in online rating and review sites is nothing to sneeze at. To wit, RateMDs was recently ranked fifth in terms of the highest share among online platforms used by consumers for choosing a provider—ahead of Twitter and just behind Instagram.

Take a look at both figures 9 and 10. One graphic shows us that about twenty-five million Americans are looking for a new primary care physician in any given twelve-month period (although they do not always find one, which is a completely separate issue). The second elucidates exactly which information sources are being used by these health seekers to find their primary care physician. Both graphics are more than ten years old and surely underestimate the actual percentage of people using the internet and the absolute number of people who are looking for a doctor today. It is really a staggering data point. Millions and millions of people are looking for a doctor at any given point in time and well over 10 percent of these people use the internet as one of their primary reference sources. Combine these two statistics and it becomes noticeably clear that the influence and power of online ratings and reviews can fundamentally shift the provision of care.

And here's what else we know: if health seekers are looking for quality signals in their choice of a provider, it is conceivable that a set of unfavorable reviews may act as that quality signal. Statistical gurus will tell you that a few bad apples in a barrel of good apples is nothing to worry about and that clinicians ought to encourage all their patients to rate them online so that there are more good reviews (i.e., apples) in the barrel to drown out the bad ones.

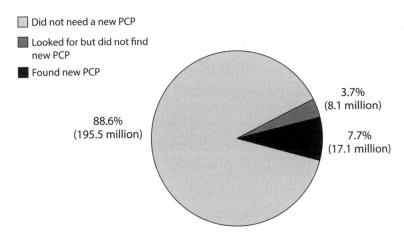

Did not need a new PCP

Looked for but did not find new PCP

Found new PCP

88.6%
(195.5 million)

3.7%
(8.1 million)

7.7%
(17.1 million)

Figure 9. US Adults Seeking and Finding New Health Care Providers in the Past 12 Months, 2007. Adapted from T. Ha Hu and R. Johanna Lauer, *Word of Mouth and Physician Referrals Still Drive Health Care Provider Choice* (Washington, DC: Center for Studying Health System Change, 2008). The Center for Studying Health System Change (HSC) was on the forefront of identifying and analyzing emerging health care trends at the community level; however, on December 31, 2013, HSC ceased operations.

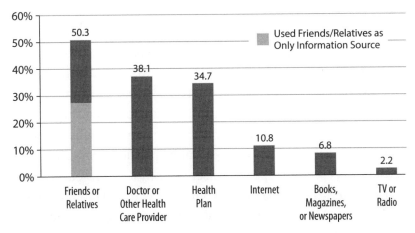

Used Friends/Relatives as Only Information Source

Figure 10. Information sources used to a select a primary care physician. Categories are not mutually exclusive; respondents could select multiple categories. T. Ha Hu and R. Johanna Lauer, *Word of Mouth and Physician Referrals Still Drive Health Care Provider Choice* (Washington, DC: Center for Studying Health System Change, 2008). The Center for Studying Health System Change was on the forefront of identifying and analyzing emerging health care trends at the community level; however, on December 31, 2013, it ceased operations.

The behavioral economists will tell you not to be that sure. They will tell you that, as we continue to shift more costs (deductibles, co-pays, etc.) to health seekers, their demands on making the right choices about their care is going to be greatly influenced by perceived value. After all, the individual health seeker's thinking is that they are paying for more and more of their care. The rallying cry for this group is going to be "bang for my buck." It is likely that the factors that have a greater perceived impact on quality will be equated with value. And that's where a couple of (hundred) reviews become important.

In an important study from the University of Michigan in September 2012, a survey asked a nationally representative sample of the US population about their knowledge and use of online ratings for selecting a physician for themselves. The results suggest that awareness of online physician ratings (65%) was lower than for other consumer goods such as cars (87%) and non–health care service providers (71%) and that this difference, for the statistical geeks, was significant. Some of this lack of awareness may actually be good news insofar as the fewer people who know about this, the greater the likelihood that there won't be an impact on their search since not knowing what one doesn't know can sometimes lead to inadvertent benefit. The bad news is that this was nine years ago, and the number is surely much higher now. In addition, among those who sought online physician ratings in the past year, 35 percent reported selecting a physician based on good ratings and 37 percent avoided a physician with bad ratings. There is some overlap between these two groups; part of the 37 percent is included in the 35 percent and vice versa. The two sets of responses are not mutually exclusive. You can, at the same time, select someone based on good ratings and avoid someone based on bad ratings. So, the authors of this article reported that 50 percent of people are influenced by online ratings. But think about the avoidance group: almost two out of every five people in this study said that they would *avoid* a physician with bad ratings. What we do not know is whether this group of health seekers is able to find a physician with good ratings to address the concern that they presumably have with their health. Which means that the negative ratings of a doctor may inadvertently drive patients away from seeking care for conditions that, unmanaged, may lead to further downstream implications involving both health deterioration and higher cost.

Interestingly, participants were also asked to consider the implications of leaving negative comments about a physician; 34 percent had concerns about their identity being disclosed, and 26 percent were concerned about the physician taking action against them.[3] Note that respondents did not voice a concern about their ratings influencing a complete stranger to seek unnecessary care or to seek care that might drive cost in the health system where, absent the review, that cost would not have been incurred. Is this because people who are posting ratings and reviews online are unaware of the impact of their actions? Or is it that they do not think there is an impact? And, so, there is a real blind spot here. Unintentional? Probably so. And, yes, we are all aware and in agreement that restaurant and vacation reviews can also result in societal waste and inefficiencies. But they are not the same. Neither of the other rating and review verticals is even remotely close to having the impact that health care reviews and ratings can have on society.

Finally, there is the tangible reality of reputational assault suffered by some very good clinicians at the hands of disgruntled patients, according to Dr. Jeffrey Segal. You'll remember the opening premise of this chapter was based on somebody spending seven to twelve minutes with you and then posting opinions on a widely viewed website. Segal, who is the founder of Medical Services Inc., is a lawyer, a board-certified neurosurgeon, and one of the US's leading authorities on medical malpractice issues, counterclaims, and internet-based assaults on reputation. In a paper that Segal published on the subject in 2009, he wrote that

> historically, if a patient were dissatisfied with care, he or she could tell his or her friends and family. The criticism was limited to a small circle of people. If the patient were injured negligently, he or she could hire an attorney to prosecute a lawsuit. The threshold for finding an attorney and prevailing posed a significant barrier for the patient achieving redress. With the Internet, if a patient is unhappy, he or she needs do little more than access a growing number of Internet physician rating sites. Such criticism can be rendered anonymously. The posts are disseminated worldwide, and once posted, the criticism rarely comes down. While transparency is a laudable goal, such sites often lack accountability.[4]

And he's not wrong. Segal proposes a solution to the current situation by suggesting that patients and providers should, at the initiation of their relationship, engage in signing a contract of mutual privacy. This mutual contract would, ostensibly, bind both parties to maintain the strictest of privacy (over and above the statutory requirements of HIPAA) and would require that the "patient agree to not post any commentary on the web about the doctor's care without the doctor's permission."[5] In the event that a posting does appear, Segal advocates contacting the site or internet service provider, filing an action for interference with a preexisting contract, launching subpoenas, and invoking breach of contract as the legal underpinning with noncompliant websites and ISPs. If, as Segal notes, the threshold for patients achieving redress was almost insurmountable back in the good old days, then surely the threshold for clinicians finding an attorney and prevailing against ISPs and websites is equally as much a significant barrier, no? Forget about the practical implications of how many doctors have the time to poke around the main rating sites to look for pernicious opinions of themselves and their services.

Let's assume a fastidious clinician can juggle a busy practice and a family while finding the time to do this. By the time the doctor finds the injurious posting, the reputational assault has happened and taken hold such that the damage to the clinician is concrete. Dwindling referrals. Canceled appointments. Loss of new patients. No number of subpoenas and "breach of contract" pleas will change the genie-is-out-of-the-bottle reality of the situation.

But is it all gloom and doom? Is there some redeeming feature of all these online ratings and reviews that might give us a sliver of hope that the system can work in good ways?

Maybe.

An online-based cross-sectional study that surveyed 2,360 physicians and other health care providers in 2015 was conducted with the aim of better understanding the likelihood that providers would implement measures to improve patient care based on these ratings. The most widely implemented quality measures were related to communication with patients (28.77%, 679/2,360), the appointment scheduling process (23.60%, 557/2,360), and office workflow (21.23%, 501/2,360). So maybe some of these reviews and ratings actually drive providers to improve care. It is one study. It is cross-sectional in nature, and I would not bet the house on it. But, directionally, this might show us that online ratings and reviews have the potential for some positive benefit in the provision of care.

We have not even begun to discuss the First Amendment complexities involved with this situation. You know the part about abridging the freedom of speech of American citizens. According to the Digital Media Law Project website,

> courts have recognized that the right to speak anonymously and
> pseudonymously is part of the First Amendment right to free speech,
> and accordingly some level of scrutiny is required before stripping an
> anonymous Internet speaker of that right. At the same time, those

harmed by unlawful anonymous speech—whether by defamation, misappropriation of trade secrets, or whatever else—also have a right to seek compensation for their injury. When considering a subpoena or other discovery request seeking to unmask a speaker, courts attempt to balance these two competing rights.[6]

While this may seem obvious as a legal precept, it reinforces that the internet is not the wild west and that rating sites may be unwitting actors in this real-world drama that is playing out.

In the end, we are in the midst of a fundamental change in the way we look at information and in the way that information is dispersed. It is not just that there are Russian bots and cyber espionage groups called Fancy Bear that impact our political elections. It is not that we have platforms such as Twitter and Facebook built for opinion sharing, ratings, and debating. It is far deeper than that. We *feel the need* to share our opinions and ratings, it seems, on absolutely everything. The food we eat. The airlines we fly. The hotels we stay at. The clothes we buy. The service we received at a retail outlet. Everything. For the most part, this rating culture and ethos we have embraced is harmless. But, in the context of health care, there is an immense challenge. How do we validate, authenticate, and allow posts of user generated content or ratings so that recipients of that information have the appropriate context? How do we ensure that people who are expressing opinions that can sway others on issues as important as health care decisions are qualified to express those opinions? How do we ensure that reputational assault is minimized while balancing the civil liberties that we hold so dear. No one, in principle, is against collecting and posting reviews or rating your doctor. And no one, in principle, wants to arrest freedom of speech. It is not any of those things.

In this connected and brave new world, we need to ask ourselves a simple question: Because we can rate something, does that mean we must? What if that rating extended to a government's response to a global pandemic?

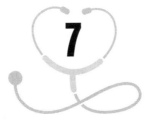

The Mother of All Nudges

Just as no building lacks an architecture, so no choice lacks a context.
—RICHARD THALER, *Nudge: Improving Decisions about Health,*
Wealth, and Happiness

During the COVID-19 pandemic, society's ability to adapt to behavioral measures was literally a matter of life and death.

This is not what Richard Thaler and Cass Sunstein, the authors of *Nudge*, one of the best-selling books on behavioral economics, had in mind. Nor Daniel Kahneman, winner of the 2002 Nobel Prize in Economic Sciences. And certainly not Steven Levitt, the coauthor of the best-selling *Freakonomics: A Rogue Economist Explores the Hidden Side of Everything*. The behavioral economics revolution was supposed to be impactful. It was going to weave its way into our everyday lives and provide a meaningful blueprint for how we could be better. Better at what, you ask. Everything. It would change the way we looked at and consumed food and how often we exercised and how we saved money. We would increase

MISUNDERSTANDING HEALTH 66

organ donation. We would smoke less. We would recycle more, thereby saving the planet. And while most in society were vaguely familiar with the concept of nudging, few paid rapt attention to it. But then COVID-19 came along in late 2019 and throughout 2020. We started paying attention to it and thought: *Wait a minute, behavioral economics was not meant to save the world, was it?*

Sunstein and Thaler define a nudge as "any aspect of the choice architecture that alters people's behavior in a predictable way, without forbidding any options or significantly changing their economic incentives."[1] We'll talk about the economic incentives part later. They are very prescriptive in their definition: nudges are not mandated, they say. Putting fruit at eye level to encourage healthy eating habits is a nudge. Banning junk food and soda pop is not.[2] Think of a nudge like the invisible hand described by Adam Smith in his eighteenth-century book *The Theory of Moral Sentiments*. Not so much in the literal sense that the unintended elements of everyday life can lead to socially desirable ends and consequences. Or that there is some unobservable force that creates a natural balance of supply and demand, which, in turn, establishes a market equilibrium. But in the more pragmatic interpretation of a nudge: guiding you in the right direction without overtly pushing you there. A gentle, but unseen, hand on your shoulder.

There is a foundational aspect of *nudge theory* that Thaler and Sunstein ask us to accept. They propose that there are significant proportions of the population who reject the paternalistic idea that the government must be involved in choice. Rather, the authors opine, there is a branch of thinking that aligns with the precept that giving people as many choices as possible and letting them choose the one they like best is the *only* way to go. Simply put, maximize the number of choices and get out of the way. Because, as Thaler and Sunstein state, these anti-paternalists believe in maximizing choice specifically because anything else is just bowing to a one-size-fits-all mentality. Of course, there are many ways to skin a cat. Providing people with choices does not mean that they all get the *same* choice. Nonetheless, at the extreme, this is the view of the anti-paternalists. But there is another aspect of nudge theory that we are asked to accept, and it is crucial to the DNA of nudge theory—the presupposition that not all people, even remotely close to all of the time, make choices in their best interest or, for that matter, even better than other people can make for them.[3]

COVID-19 illustrates my point perfectly. We saw a slew of behavioral health nudges emanating from hundreds of countries around the world that were, literally, a matter of life and death. Governments placed that proverbial hand on our societal shoulder and asked us to stay at home. To wash our hands frequently and often. To keep two meters apart from one another when we do go out. To sneeze into our elbow. To social distance. To shelter in place. To not shake hands. To not hoard basic necessities.

But remember the underlying principle that I said I would come back to later. Nudges must not change an individual's economic incentives. With COVID-19, it is not obviously clear if this is a problem. Of course, we have changed the economic incentives of millions of people but not through nudges. Closing down an entire economy so that there is no commercial activity is not a nudge. This is the public health equivalent of banning junk food and soda. The actual nudging has not really changed anyone's economic incentive in the strictest definition. Some will argue that the very nature of social distancing is a nudge that affects an individual's economic incentives. But it is not really. In many parts of the world, even if you do not social distance, there is barely anything open. Most people cannot go earn money or sell their wares or spend to their heart's content anyway. And the reason that you cannot do those things is not due to a nudge. It is because in many countries around the world, governments have mandated that many businesses must close. They have applied the "junk food and soda" principle to the economy.

These nudges are the right principles for all countries to adopt if your goal is to put public health first and everything else second. There is some debate as to whether that is truly the goal of every nation but, that aside, the important question (if public health is the primary goal) is how we make these nudges "sticky" without mandating citizens to do them, without rolling tanks into the streets and imposing curfews and martial law. After all, when the government *forces* you to do something, this is no longer a behavioral nudge. Just ask the citizens of Wuhan who, by all accounts, were subjected to literal house arrest for months and months and, at the same time, tracked by cell phone apps and drones to ensure that social distancing mandates were met.

Underpinning this large question around "stickiness" are some of the smaller, more nuanced questions to consider: Does expected utility theory still hold true in the case of a global pandemic? In other words, do decisions made under conditions of uncertainty about expected outcomes (becoming infected) and the hope that people behave rationally still apply when everyone has the same uncertainty? Maybe everyone doesn't have the same uncertainty about expected outcomes. Maybe some people know more than others. In which case, information asymmetry may affect people's behavior during this pandemic in ways that have not been well captured to date.

Expected utility theory is originally credited to Daniel Bernoulli, a Swiss mathematician, who, in the eighteenth century, espoused the view that "the price of the item is dependent only on the thing itself and is equal for everyone; the utility, however, is dependent on the particular circumstances of the person making the estimate. Thus, there is no doubt that a gain of one thousand ducats is more significant to a pauper than to a rich man though both gain the same amount."[4] In other words, the value of a decision made under uncertainty is not a function of the price of the good but, rather, a function of the benefit and satisfaction that it brings to the individual.

There are four key axioms of expected utility theory that I will not dive into in any depth, save to mention them (completeness, transitivity, independence, and continuity) and to express that they all involve some aspect of the number of choices available and the preference for these choices when making a decision. What does all this have to do with COVID-19? Well, there are tenets in health policy that focus on calculating health utilities where we assign a value of "0" to being dead and a value of "1" to being in the best imaginable health state. We can implement various techniques to calculate an individual's utility for a particular health state by using the principles of the standard gamble, the time trade-off, and other such utility measures, with each involving a varying degree of uncertainty. At its core, the challenge with expected utility theory in the context of COVID-19 and the idea of making decisions under uncertainty is that conventional utility theory would suggest that there is an intermediate health outcome or health state against which you are gambling, or trading off. But with COVID-19, we do not know what that intermediate state is. Or, more to the point, it varies so wildly that it is nearly impossible to gauge accurately. Is the intermediate health state a high fever and hacking cough that leaves you exhausted but, after recovery, able to resume a normal life? Or is the intermediate health state one of being admitted to a hospital, ending up in the intensive care unit, and ultimately on mechanical ventilation? Or is it something in-between?

What about the concept of externalities and their importance in the context of public health during the COVID-19 pandemic of 2020, which should not be lost on us? Today, this concept, intertwined with the larger idea of nudges, is truer than it has ever been in modern memory. Everything that everyone does has an impact on everyone's health. Externalities are the new normal. The notion that *your* behavior has an impact on *my* health has never been clearer. From a strict economic sense, we define externalities as scenarios in which the effect of producing or consuming a good or service imposes costs or benefits on others, which are not reflected in the prices charged for those goods and services being provided.[5] In the world of public health and health policy, the practical implication of this definition is that sometimes the things people do have an effect on other people's health. If those effects are positive effects, we deem the situation to have created a positive externality, and, similarly, if the effect is negative, then we acknowledge a negative externality. Let's briefly look at two such examples. Suppose for a moment that I get an annual influenza vaccine, or flu shot (which in the context of COVID-19 is an extremely germane example). While the vaccine largely protects me from getting the flu, it also protects you, to some degree, from contracting the flu virus from me. Hence, the act of my getting a flu vaccine grants you and others in my circle a level of herd immunity. You accrue some level of protection against a virus because I have vaccinated myself. This is an example of a positive externality—a benefit extended to you because of my behavior. Conversely, let's assume that I smoke cigarettes and that we live under the same roof. The secondhand smoke from my smoking habit may deliver health outcomes to you such as respiratory infections or an increased risk of cardiovascular disease. In this situation, my behavior inflicts a negative externality on you and others who live in the same household—namely, that, as a result of my behavior, you are now at increased risk of illness.

That externalities are an everyday part of health care is not a new revelation. It is (always) the how that matters the most. How do we get more people to engage in positive externality behaviors and less often in negative externality behaviors. In most situations, the individual and societal benefits of increasing positive externalities or decreasing negative externalities are immense (imagine if everyone got vaccinated or quit smoking). The schools of thought on how best to motivate such obvious positive externalities have frequently centered on subsidies/cost-sharing and free distribution. Let's give away insecticide-treated nets to prevent malaria or make vaccines free at the point of care. Uptake and usage are guaranteed to be massive, no? Sadly, this is not the case.

The stark reality is that giving away free things or imposing nominal user fees is not the sole determinant of whether people engage in a specific health-related behavior. Individuals must value the good or service at a level tied to the externality. In the case of cost-sharing or subsidies, we must be careful that the amount we charge does not selectively screen out those individuals who place a high value on the good or service but who can afford it the least. This will undoubtedly be one of the major challenges with producing and distributing a COVID-19 vaccine. How will we ensure that poorer countries have access to the vaccine considering what is sure to be an out-of-reach price point.

Public education is also needed to truly motivate some of these behavioral tendencies—often a challenge in jurisdictions with low literacy levels where a basic understanding of important health behaviors is fleeting at best and where government mistrust is rampant. In the mind's eye when we think about this idea conceptually, we immediately think about sub-Saharan Africa or the villages of India. But, perhaps, with the anti-vaxxers frothing at the mouth during COVID-19, this is an even bigger challenge in the developed world where health literacy and government mistrust are no less of an issue but are complemented by both technological cunning and deep pockets that allow for misinformation and the fomenting of troublesome anti-vaccine opinions.[6] We must consider access to health care as a critical component in the overall context of improving externality-related behaviors. Perhaps a patient wants to get a vaccine but does not have reliable transport to get to their health care provider. In addition, nudging people's behaviors to increase positive externalities through a financial mechanism that involves no risk for the patient may lead to a low willingness-to-pay in the future. After all, price does signal quality, which also affects perceived value. Certainly, we must consider that a free-at-the-point-of-care model or high subsidy levels do have implications for other programs within the health budget and diminish some level of reimbursement or cost recovery that may have potentially been (re)allocated elsewhere. Externalities are critically important components of our health system. We do not always refer to them by their technical name, but we pay attention to them because of their potential massive impact on public health. As we turn to behavioral approaches to help solve crises like the COVID-19 pandemic, let's keep in mind that improving my health outcomes by relying on your behavior change is tricky business.

Another critical topic to ensure nudges are actually adopted is health literacy. Telling some people to quarantine and others to isolate themselves is fine and well. But do people know what each means? Are they able to distinguish between the two? Herd immunity is not an easy concept to understand during the best of times. Does everyone have the same understanding of this concept? As a cornerstone of nudge adoption, how do we actually address inequalities in health literacy? We're not going to eradicate entrenched problems that have plagued us for decades, but ensuring that we communicate in simple language and in multiple languages to reach citizens of all mother tongues is a global imperative. Why do I refer to it as a global imperative? Because research shows that people who are better informed about their health status are more likely to have better outcomes. Differences between high health literacy levels and low health literacy levels have been consistently associated with increased hospitalizations, greater emergency care use, lower use of mammography, lower receipt of influenza vaccine, poorer ability to demonstrate taking medications appropriately, poorer ability to interpret labels and health messages, and, among seniors, poorer overall health status and higher mortality in those individuals who have lower health literacy. In the context of the COVID-19 pandemic, with the possible exception of mammography use, all of these associations between health literacy and outcomes are strikingly important.

Another reason nudges depend on health literacy is that there are groups of people who, by virtue of their young age, lack of underlying comorbidities, or prioritization of other needs above health, do not understand the value of the public health recommendations. They choose to "free ride" on the actions of others or to deliberately spread misinformation for personal and economic gain.

> Health literacy might help people to grasp the reasons behind the recommendations and reflect on outcomes of their various possible actions. However, taking social responsibility, thinking beyond personal interests, and understanding how people make choices—aspects such as ethical viewpoints and behavioural insights—should also be considered within the toolbox of health literacy. Solidarity and social responsibility should not only be accounted for by the general population and decision makers, but also by those individuals who produce and share misleading and false information about SARS-CoV-2.[7]

Abel and McQueen also underscore the misinformation aspect of COVID-19 and its relationship to health literacy: "What is different with situations like COVID-19 is that we live in an age when expectations about mastering health—and here that means specifically, controlling risks of a deadly infectious disease—are higher than ever. These advanced expectations meet with another unique condition: never in human history has there been such an abundance of health information available from numerous more or less trustworthy sources."[8]

A last critical issue is the use of the internet to find online health information. Specifically, how the practice of online health information–seeking behavior can adversely affect access to care, treatment decisions, and allocation of scarce resources. The COVID-19 pandemic of 2020 heightened my concerns in this regard with a veritable deluge of misinformation spewed forth on a daily basis (particularly as it relates to treatment options for combating this virus). In an *MIT Technology Review* article, Karen Hao delved into this issue, and what she found was alarming. Researchers studied more than two hundred million tweets discussing coronavirus or COVID-19 since January 2020. They used machine-learning and network analysis techniques to identify which accounts were spreading disinformation and which were most likely bots or cyborgs (accounts run jointly by bots and humans). Through the analysis, they identified more than one hundred types of inaccurate COVID-19 stories and found that not only were bots gaining traction and accumulating followers, but they accounted for 82 percent of the top fifty and 62 percent of the top one thousand influential retweeters. The influence of each account was calculated to reflect the number of followers it reached as well as the number of followers its followers reached.[9]

Set aside what we discussed earlier about using health literacy not only to enhance the understanding of important public health recommendations so that people minimize their risk of being infected but also to show those spreading misinformation that their actions have a tremendous toll on human life. How do we counter the dissemination of dangerous and nonscientific data, period? Whether or not there is a health literacy link. More important, how can we nudge tech companies to limit misinformation, which is proving to have found an incredibly fertile host on the internet? We have seen the ugly face of misinformation in political elections and tabloid fodder. Even in those situations where no direct human life is on the line, many people are incapable of distinguishing between high-accuracy and low-accuracy information. Now imagine a complex disease with complex etiology and tortuous mandates, recommendations, and requirements.

With millions of people infected and hundreds of thousands, unfortunately, dead, the COVID-19 pandemic of 2020 has changed the way we conduct our lives forever. There is no doubt about this. The use of behavioral nudging and its incorporation into public policy is here. But, in its current format as a blunt instrument of direction to millions of people, are we using it the right way? What is the right way? Does anyone agree on what that looks like? What if nudges could be used to impact some of the obvious social determinants of health that so clearly impact population health?

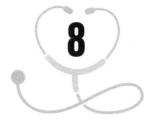

Your Health Is about More Than Just Your Health

He who has health, has hope; and he who has hope, has everything.
—Thomas Carlyle

Your health is about way more than just your health.

A bit of a mind twister, no? We all know this intuitively, but we never really internalize it the way policy makers are forced to commit this mantra to memory. Most people do not believe that their health is only a function of their genes or that the entire sum of their health is neatly compartmentalized in the physical exam and the lab results they get once a year. I am quite confident that most people realize that genetics are an incredibly important predictor of disease. I am also equally confident that these same people realize other factors also contribute to disease, illness, and morbidity.

In the everyday parlance of health policy wonks and epidemiology geeks, we call these other factors *social determinants of health* and include educational attainment, income, nutritional support, and residential and racial segregation. According to the World Health Organization, "the social determinants of health are the conditions in which people are born, grow, live, work and age. These circumstances are shaped by the distribution of money, power, and resources at global, national, and local levels. The social determinants of health are mostly responsible for health inequities—the unfair and avoidable differences in health status seen within and between countries."[1] Note that the definition includes the term *health inequities* and not *health inequalities*. This is a nuanced but important distinction. Another important term is *fairness*. Overcoming health inequality means making things the same for everyone, whereas overcoming health inequities means making things *fair* for everyone. A really good idea of this concept is presented in figure 11. When we attempt to

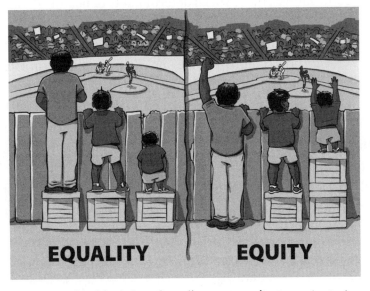

Figure 11. Graphical depiction of equality versus equity. Interaction Institute for Social Change. Artist: Angus Maguire.

solve for inequality, we give everyone the same tools and re-sources, thereby leaving the relative gap between them the same. When we attempt to solve for inequity, we consider the individual's starting point and close the gap between them so that, presumably, things are fairer.

By providing a vaccine to everyone for a nominal amount of money (i.e., a user fee) at the point of care, we make things equal. Everyone pays the same. But the gap between the haves and have-nots has not changed. Those who have trouble paying for health care services and treatments through out-of-pocket payments will still have trouble. By charging only those above a certain income threshold or, conversely, subsidizing those below another threshold, we now change the dynamic. We have created fairness. Individuals in society are charged on their ability to pay instead of a flat fee across the board.

Why do we struggle so much with implementing programs required to address these social determinants of health? Perhaps Taylor et al. have hit on an important feature in their summary of the peer-reviewed literature on the subject from 2016. In this review, the authors summarized the impact of investments in social services or investments in integrated models of health care and social services on health outcomes and health care spending. Of thirty-nine papers that met criteria for inclusion in the review, thirty-two (82%) reported some significant positive effects on either health outcomes ($N = 20$), health care costs ($N = 5$), or both ($N = 7$). Despite this strong association, they surmise that the problem with wider adoption of these programs may be due to *wrong pocket problem*.

> The savings that accompany health improvements do not accrue to the investor . . . many social service interventions (e.g., income support, housing) generate positive health outcomes, yet social service sectors receive little if any reward for their contribution to the

creation of health in the population. Similarly . . . a health care organization that contributes to a person's health does not reap the full social benefit from those health improvements. Thus, the wrong pocket problem discourages cross-sector collaboration when in fact the literature reviewed here suggests a high degree of mutual dependence and potential reward from coordinated health care and social services.[2]

So, there you have it. In simple terms, this is a what's-in-it-for-me issue that is not altogether an uncommon occurrence in wider public policy.

It is odd though and counterintuitive when you think about it. McCullough[3] recently published on the subject of better understanding public health's wrong pocket problem, and he elucidates work that shows that for every $1 invested in public health departments, there was a staggering return of $67 to $88 of benefits to society.[4] Other studies, he points out, have estimated smaller but still positive returns on public health spending, too.[5] McCullough goes on to state that "in theory, health stakeholders, policymakers, taxpayers, and even private investors would flock to finance investments with such positive returns on investment—yet public health spending in the U.S. has fallen as proportion of total health spending beginning around 2000 and in inflation-adjusted terms since the Great Recession."[6] A perplexing paradox to say the least.

We attempt to address inequities in health and make things fairer for everyone. But we are saddled with the knowledge that making things fairer does not galvanize society into action. Inertia governs for many reasons. First, there is the temporal nature of the problem. Making improvements in public health and reducing inequities is an undertaking of, usually, years and years of work. The money is spent today, and the benefit accrues years in the future, which prevents those who spend from seeing the benefits of their investment. It also prevents those who accrue the benefits from drawing a straight line to the spending that affected their bottom line. This leads to the natural follow-on problem, which, of course, is the unavoidable disincentive on the part of beneficiaries to unilaterally invest in public health because they still stand to benefit regardless of whether they decide to invest their own resources.[7]

As much as your genetics and your lifestyle factors play a critical role in your health, social determinants of health can be directly attributable to hundreds of thousands of deaths. Galea et al. actually calculated the deaths attributable to each of the social factors in the United States in a single year (2000) and compared them to deaths from three of the leading disease killers in the United States (see tables 4 and 5).[8] It is staggering to think about and eye-opening when you look at some of the deeper statistics on each one of these dimensions. The caveat is always the same: We can argue and debate about the methodological choices and statistical techniques used to calculate the results in any study. We will always find alternative ways to have either set up the original study design or interpreted the results. This is a fact. Short of egregious data manipulation or something similar, this should not be our focus on this topic. We need to look at these data (particularly since it is nonrandomized data) for what they are: directional in nature and potentially hypothesis generating or, as some might

Table 4. Deaths attributable to social factors in the US in 2000

Social Factor	Number of Deaths in US, 2000
Low education	244,526
Racial segregation	175,520
Low social support	161,522
Individual-level poverty	133,250
Income inequality	119,208
Area-level poverty	39,330

Source: Galea et al. (2011).

Table 5. Deaths from disease in the US in 2000

Disease	Number of Deaths in US, 2000
Acute myocardial infarction	192,898
Cerebrovascular disease	167,661
Lung cancer	155,521

Source: Galea et al. (2011).

argue, hypothesis validating. With this out of the way, let's acknowledge the limitations in this type of analysis and that these
numbers should be regarded through the filter of a relationship
between A and B, which requires us to pay attention and to be informed. And this is certainly true of the data around deaths attributable to social factors as the authors themselves acknowledge. We must pay attention to this. There is most certainly an
overlap here. Deaths attributable to low education are, of course,
associated with individual-level poverty. Deaths attributable to
individual-level poverty are most certainly linked to income inequality. But directionally, this is telling us something important
that we have all known for years but is often not juxtaposed next
to such stark numbers: your overall health and its future outlook
are most certainly not only about your genetics; there is a level of
morbidity and mortality associated with social determinants of
health that requires urgent intervention.

The Robert Wood Johnson Foundation conducted a series of
analyses on these social determinants of health and found that
residential segregation (i.e., where you live) has a major effect on
overall health outcomes (figure 12). Within a radius of nine to seventeen Metro stops (ten to thirty miles) in Washington, DC, the
life span of individuals can change by as much as nine years.[9] The
cheeky way of thinking about this is that our zip codes may mean
as much to our health status as our genetic codes. Think about this
for a moment. Your life span can be almost ten years shorter simply

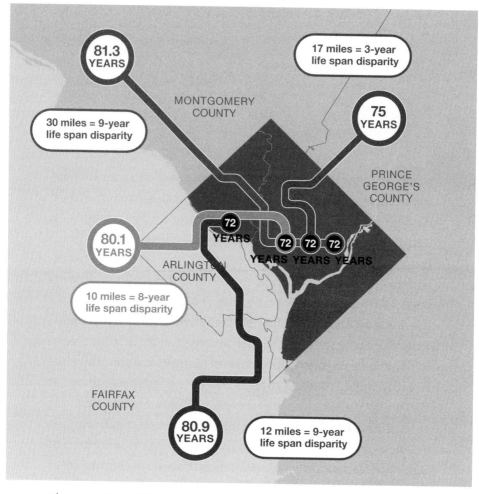

Figure 12. Map of Washington, DC, showing discrepancy in life expectancy along various Metro lines. Robert Wood Johnson Foundation, *Overcoming Obstacles to Health* (Washington, DC: Robert Wood Johnson Foundation, 2008), www.commission onhealth.org.

based on where you live. This is not a comparison between life spans in sub-Saharan Africa and North America. This is a comparison between life spans in the same city.

Don't believe it? More than a decade ago, the Robert Wood Johnson Foundation, which is the largest philanthropy dedicated solely to health in the United States, published a report entitled *Overcoming Obstacles to Health*. This report really laid it on the line. Racial segregation creates natural health inequities in everyday ways that many of us take for granted, such as "living in a neighborhood where fresh produce is not sold or where tobacco and alcohol advertising on billboards are common, or having a workplace without breastfeeding accommodations. Similarly, receiving recommended medical care may depend on factors like living near medical offices and clinics, having access to transportation and childcare."[10] Think about the racially segregated neighborhood where you live. Think about how most of us do not realize that these natural barriers to good health are built into these neighborhoods.

And the graphical portrayal of health disparities based on income and education are just as stark (figures 13 and 14).

These social determinants of health should not be viewed in isolation from one another. A lower education has the potential to cause enough damage to an individual's health simply by virtue of our knowledge about the association between educational attainment and health literacy. The lower the number of years of total schooling, the lower the overall health literacy score. The lower the score, the worse the outcomes. We have known for many years that differences in health literacy levels have been consistently associated with increased hospitalizations, greater emergency care use, lower use of mammography, lower receipt of influenza vaccine, poorer ability to demonstrate taking medications appropriately, poorer ability to interpret labels and health messages, and, among seniors, poorer overall health status and higher mortality.[11]

There is also that interplay between determinants that I referred to earlier and the realization that many of these social factors are not isolated contributors to health inequities. A lower education also affects where you live. Why? Because your level of education undoubtedly impacts the type of job you get, which

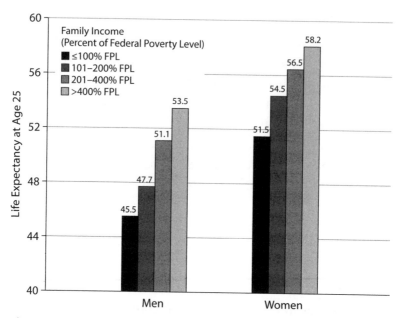

Figure 13. Family Income and Health. Prepared for the Robert Wood Johnson Foundation by the Center on Social Disparities in Health at the University of California, San Francisco; and Norman Johnson, U.S. Bureau of the Census. National Longitudinal Mortality Study, 1988–1998.

impacts how much you earn. And how much you earn determines how much you can afford to pay for rent or a mortgage. If you cannot afford to pay a higher rent or get the mortgage you need to live in a desirable neighborhood, chances are you may end up in a neighborhood that negatively impacts your health. Because you have a high school education instead of college degree and because you could not get that high-paying job, you cannot afford a car. Because you cannot afford a car, you have to rely on public transportation to get to your medical appointments, which are all the way across town. That is if you can even make it to your medical appointments because your low(er) income job has forced you to live in a less-than-desirable neighborhood where reliable and accessible childcare is a challenge. Of course, this is important

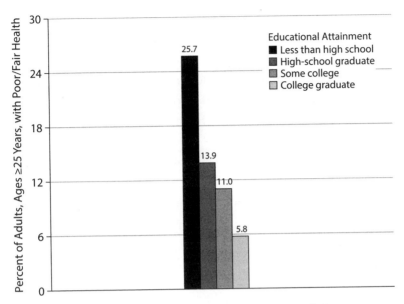

Figure 14. Education and health. Prepared for the Robert Wood Johnson Foundation by the Center on Social Disparities in Health at the University of California, San Francisco; National Health Interview Survey, 2001–2005, age-adjusted.

because you need someone to watch the kids after school so that you can get to your medical appointment. I am being purposefully deliberate about connecting the dots for you. Not because I doubt your ability to see the complex connectivity between the various social determinants of health. But because by spelling it out in such a blunt fashion, it forces us to confront the magnitude of the problem.

We can hope that one out of every thousand children are able to break out of this cycle of despair. But those numbers do not move the needle. We can hope that a visionary body of lawmakers ascends to office with a bold courage that addresses what is needed twenty-five years down the road. But, as the saying goes, "hope is not a strategy." We need investment in the form of public-private partnerships. We need drastic measures over a generation that impact more than the lucky few. And we need to track the outcomes longitudinally to show that they work. We need free housing for socioeconomically disadvantaged people for a fixed, but meaningful, period of time. We need free schooling through university. We need income equality policies that allow the disadvantaged a tangible mechanism to close the gap between their income and the median income. We need free childcare and free public transportation for those who are most in need.

But what we need the most is to remember the axiom epitomized by Thomas Jefferson: "There is nothing more unequal than the equal treatment of unequal people."

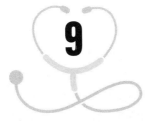

9

Needle in a Haystack

God hath given you one face, and you make yourself another.

—WILLIAM SHAKESPEARE, *Hamlet*

Health screening programs seem so simple in their objectives.

To ensure that we're all on the same page, the widely accepted definition of *screening* centers on the application of a simple test to asymptomatic persons to classify them as likely or unlikely to have a disease.[1] Screening is not a diagnostic test. In other words, a screening test will not tell you whether you have a disease or an illness. All we are really trying to do is find out whether someone is likely to become sick before it is too late to start some meaningful treatment. How, theoretically, could early detection of disease not be beneficial?

How is it possible that taking asymptomatic people and classifying them as likely or unlikely to have a disease be anything other than good and how could treatment *before* symptoms develop not be better than treatment *after* symptoms develop? Surprisingly, though, we struggle with screening programs, and the answers to these questions are not as straightforward as they may seem. As with many issues in health care and health policy, we struggle because we have conflicting actors who all bring different viewpoints to this debate. We struggle with screening programs for a variety of other reasons, too—most notably of which is that screening programs have led to increases in the diagnosis of diseases but have not necessarily led to decreases in mortality. And that is the real reason we struggle with screening programs: because they are not always successful by the standards we measure success in health care—mortality reduction.

Recently, the United States Preventive Services Task Force (USPSTF) sought public opinion on prostate cancer screening and reviewed the evidence available to them. Their draft conclusion was that for men ages fifty-five to sixty-nine, the decision to receive prostate specific antigen–based screening should be between the clinician and the patient, include a complete understanding of all potential harms as well as benefits, and incorporate the patient's values and preferences (C grade) (table 6). For men seventy and older, the USPSTF recommends against PSA-based screening because the potential benefits do not outweigh the harms (D grade).[2] Clearly, this is an overt admission by a panel of experts that, based on a systematic review of the evidence, there is, at best, no more than a moderate level of certainty that the net benefit of screening is small. In fact, in certain age groups of men, the harms outweigh the benefits.

What do we need for a successful screening program? Well, we need a suitable disease. This may sound odd, but not all diseases lend themselves to screening. Certainly, orphan and ultra-orphan diseases are not suitable for screening programs. Although orphan and ultra-orphan diseases have serious outcomes (including high mortality rates), their prevalence is too low. The number of people who are at risk for these diseases at any given point in time is not high enough. This is central to the implementation of a screening

Table 6. Grade, definitions, and suggestions for practice

Grade	Definition	Suggestions for Practice
A	The USPSTF recommends the service. There is high certainty that the net benefit is substantial.	Offer or provide this service.
B	The USPSTF recommends the service. There is high certainty that the net benefit is moderate or there is moderate certainty that the net benefit is moderate to substantial.	Offer or provide this service.
C	The USPSTF recommends selectively offering or providing this service to individual patients based on professional judgment and patient preferences. There is at least moderate certainty that the net benefit is small.	Offer or provide this service for selected patients depending on individual circumstances.
D	The USPSTF recommends against the service. There is moderate or high certainty that the service has no net benefit or that the harms outweigh the benefits.	Discourage the use of this service.
I Statement	The USPSTF concludes that the current evidence is insufficient to assess the balance of benefits and harms of the service. Evidence is lacking, of poor quality, or conflicting, and the balance of benefits and harms cannot be determined.	Read the clinical considerations section of USPSTF recommendation statement. If the service is offered, patients should understand the uncertainty about the balance of benefits and harms.

Note: USPSTF = United States Preventive Services Task Force.

program because we need enough people at risk for the disease to justify the cost and required resource allocation for such a screening program to be implemented.

Diseases best suited for screening must also be detectable in the preclinical phase, which is a fancy way of saying that there are two important anchor points in the entire screening process: the biological onset of the disease and the detection of the disease by symptoms. The time between the biological onset of the disease (say, breast cancer) and the detection of the disease by symptoms (say, a lump) is known as the *detectable preclinical phase*. In this stage, a disease should and can be detectable by screen and an individual should and can be screened—only during this time. As a reminder, we need to screen only during this detectable preclinical phase because well, for one thing, you cannot screen for a disease before its actual biological onset. Second, you cannot screen for a disease after it has become detectable by symptomology because, at that point, the individual being screened is no longer asymptomatic and, technically, you are no longer screening. You are now in the phase of treating active disease. So, there is this critical and, in some diseases, narrow window of opportunity for screening.

Imperatively, a suitable disease must be one in which treatment before symptoms emerge is better than treatment after symptoms emerge. Otherwise, the costs to the system and the burden to the patient render the screening inconsequential. Good examples of screening programs where the early detection, diagnosis, and treatment have favorable outcomes are glaucoma, hypertension, and breast cancer. Scenarios in which early screening makes little difference are diseases such as ovarian and pancreatic cancers. It is not that we do not want to detect these diseases early. It is that these diseases are highly fatal, and early detection before symptoms develop has little impact on mortality.

What else matters in the screening of disease? Let us assume that we have got our suitable disease identified. Now we need a suitable test. A suitable test is characterized by its simplicity and ease of administration, its low cost, and the fact that it is well-tolerated by the patient (i.e., not too invasive).[3] Mostly, a suitable test must be valid. The test must do what it is intended to do. It must have high *sensitivity* and *specificity*. If an individual tests

Blood Pressure		Hypertension		
		Yes	No	
	+	175	1,283	1,458
	–	65	77,650	77,715
		240	78,933	79,173

Figure 15. Fictitious example of screening for hypertension.

positive, the individual should truly have the disease, and if the individual tests negative, the individual should be disease free.

Using blood pressure to screen for hypertension illustrates the interplay between sensitivity and specificity. The sensitivity of blood pressure to screen for hypertension would be the proportion of people who screen positive over the total number of people who have hypertension. In this fictitious example depicted in figure 15, the sensitivity of a blood pressure test to screen for hypertension would be 175/240, or 73 percent, and we could reasonably say that the probability of this screening test correctly identifying diseased subjects was 73 percent.[4] The specificity of the blood pressure screening program for hypertension would be the proportion of people who screen negative over the total number of people who do not have hypertension, which would work out to 77,650/78,933, or 98 percent. Again, we could say that the probability of this screening test correctly identifying nondiseased subjects was 98 percent. So, we would conclude that this screening test was excellent at identifying individuals who did not have hypertension but that it missed 27 percent of individuals who did have hypertension. Why am I bothering with the finer points of sensitivity and specificity? Because this aspect of screening is critical. You can have the right disease, the impact of screening on mortality can be high, and the screening program can be implemented in a cost-effective manner with low friction for individuals, but if the test does not do what it is supposed to do—which is to identify the right individuals who are likely to get the disease so that early intervention can reduce mortality—then nothing else matters.

But before I move on, there is another important aspect to this whole discussion that needs to be elucidated. And I will use a different example from hypertension to distinguish between sensitivity and specificity and what I am about to shed light on.

Suppose for a moment that there is a screening test to predict the likelihood of suffering a broken arm and that you are screened for a broken arm. Let us say that our screening test gives us a positive result. The test predicts that you have a broken arm. We order an X-ray, and it confirms the positive result of our screening test, that you, indeed, have a broken arm. This, in the parlance of epidemiology and, specifically, decision science theory, is what we call a *true positive*. You screened positive for a disease or ailment and you truly do have the disease or ailment. Let us look at the flip side. Suppose now that you are screened for a broken arm. Let us say that our screening test gives us a negative result. The test predicts that you will not have a broken arm. We order an X-ray, and it confirms the negative result of our screening test, that you, indeed, do not have a broken arm. This is what we call a *true negative*. You screened negative for a disease or ailment, and you truly do not have the disease or ailment.

		Broken Arm		
		Yes	No	
Screening test for broken arm	+	175	1,283	1,458
	−	65	77,650	77,715
		240	78,933	79,173

Figure 16. Fictitious example of false positive and false negative in broken arm scenario.

In both instances, there is something obvious that has occurred: the screening test was correct. In one scenario, it said you had an ailment and you did. In another, it said you did not have an ailment and you did not.

In the true positive scenario, since the test was correct, painkillers are prescribed and perhaps a cast or splint is placed on your arm and you go home. The costs incurred are in line with the resources delivered. In the true negative scenario, since the test was also correct, nothing is prescribed, and no casts or splints are placed. The costs incurred are, too, in line with the resources delivered.

But what happens when the test is wrong?

What happens when the test delivers a *false positive*? What happens when the test says you have a broken arm and you do not (see top right number in 2 × 2 grid in figure 16)? Well, let's think about this for a second. If I am treated for a broken arm, and I do not really have one, then the system incurs costs. I see the doctor for follow-up visits. I take time off work. I get a cast and painkillers when I do not need them. Maybe I suffer from some adverse events due to the painkillers that I never needed. And maybe I suffer from some stress and anxiety.

What happens when the test delivers a *false negative*? What happens when the test comes back negative and says that you do not have a broken arm, but you really do (see lower left number in 2 × 2 grid in figure 16)? In this case, you may not incur splint and painkiller costs at the point of diagnosis, but you incur the cost of ongoing pain and suffering, the cost of this untreated morbidity, lost productivity, time off work, and maybe some downstream effect of not being properly diagnosed in the first place (i.e., more advanced disease requiring expensive intervention that would not have been necessary had your disease been caught in the first place).

This is where health care gets really, really tricky. We tend to focus on the costs we incur in the patients who *have* disease. And we disregard costs for patients in whom we find no disease. But the false positives and false negatives in health care drive costs that nobody accounts for. Ever. When a hospital gets its annual budget, the government does not give it a few extra million dollars to treat patients who do not really have disease. The government does not announce some sort of slush fund for hospitals to dip into to treat patients that were screened as false positives. And, inversely, nobody puts together a budget that has a buffer for taking care of patients who have disease that we never realized was there in the first place. We do not have the luxury of accessing health care dollars for the false negatives. It just does not work that way. It is all one big pot of money. Screening programs while immensely valuable can also be inefficient. Yes, not every disease or ailment falls into this neat little false positive or false negative category by virtue of what I discussed earlier in this chapter. It is hard to quantify the extent of these costs—it is conceivable that they are a drop in the bucket. And perhaps, most germanely, there is no obvious way to eliminate the problem of false positives and false negatives. Medicine is not perfect. It makes mistakes. And that is OK. But it is worth pointing out that even these honest mistakes cost money.

Now back to screening at a broad level. We have got a suitable disease and a suitable test. We put them together to develop a program and ask ourselves whether the program is, indeed, feasible and effective. Can we do it? Does it matter if we do it?

On the question of feasibility, we need to know whether we can identify enough cases and whether those cases can be reliably moved forward to diagnosis and treatment. As obvious as it sounds, the feasibility of a screening program only works if we take people who screened positive and then provide them with follow-up care. While I will not spend a lot of time on it, the feasibility of a screening program is also contingent on total cost and the cost-effectiveness per case identified. This is an obvious comment, but someone needs to find the money. We must consider the yield of the screening program as well through mechanisms such as the positive and negative predictive values and disease prevalence. In other words, what proportion of those people who screened positive for a disease actually have preclinical disease. Similarly, what proportion of those people who screened negative for a disease actually do not have preclinical disease.[5] In our hypertension and broken arm examples, the positive predictive value of both of these screening programs would be the output of 175/1,458, which is 12 percent. For those who may be wondering, this 12 percent value is not terribly impressive. The usefulness of this screening program, as a function of its positive predictive value, is low. What this says in lay terms is that, of all the people who were screened for our disease, our screening test was only able to detect disease correctly in 12 percent of screened individuals. But that is because the prevalence of hypertension in our screened population was very low (175/79,173, or 0.22%). If we had chosen a different population to screen, our screening program yield would be much better. If we want to get the most value out of our screening program, it is abundantly clear that we ought to target a subset of the population likely to have a higher prevalence of disease, and we should not screen individuals who are very unlikely to be diseased.[6]

On the question of effectiveness, the central point is about actual outcomes. If we have a suitable disease and a suitable and feasible test, but we do not pick up early disease or impact survival/mortality, then we can say the screening program is not effective. While impact on survival and/or mortality is a nice, neat way to categorize the effectiveness of a screening program, our evaluation of a screening program's effectiveness is greatly influenced by potential bias. In an observational data set, we could be faced with a common problem known as *volunteer bias* in which those who volunteer, or self-select, for screening could be systematically different than those who do not volunteer in ways associated with the outcome. Maybe the volunteers are healthier and just part of a population segment that we call the *worried well*. Or, conversely, maybe the volunteers are at higher risk.

Then there is a serious bias that we must consider, known as *lead-time bias*. Here is how this works: by definition, a screening program advances the date of diagnosis of a disease in an asymptomatic person than would have naturally occurred without the screening. Make sense? If I screen a woman for breast cancer and it turns out she does have the disease, I have advanced her diagnosis by a factor of time that would not have otherwise occurred if she had just been diagnosed on the basis of observable symptoms such as a lump in her breast. This factor of time is known as the *lead time*. And if we are not careful in our analysis of this patient subpopulation of screened individuals, it can appear as though they have survived longer than nonscreened individuals only because their diagnosis date was pushed back.[7]

Here is a real example of that.[8]

- A randomized trial was conducted to evaluate the effectiveness of a new screening program for colon cancer.
- Among those whose cancers were *detected by the screening program,* the average age at diagnosis was fifty-four years and average age at death was sixty years: thus, the average survival from diagnosis to death was six years.
- For those *detected by clinical symptoms,* average age at diagnosis was fifty-six years and average age at death was sixty years: thus, the average survival from diagnosis to death was four years.
- The investigators reported a statistically significant two-year *increase in survival* from colon cancer associated with screening.
- What is wrong with this picture?

In this rudimentary example, it is clear to see that both groups died at age sixty. There was no increase in survival in the screened group as compared to the clinical symptom group. What we can say with certainty is that the only increase that occurred is the increase of time that the screened group knew they had colon cancer.

So, there you have it. It is not easy. Screening is not appropriate for all diseases and screening programs cost a lot. And they have to be designed to be easy for the public to participate in. We have to be careful about false positives and negatives as well as biases that can prevent us from incorrectly evaluating the screening program's utility. Despite all of these challenges and considerations, perhaps the greatest benefit of screening programs is that we get people in the health care system on a regular and routine basis. People who otherwise would not be seeing their doctors are now doing so. And maybe this unintended consequence of screening is how we ought to be looking at it. Or maybe another unintended consequence is that we are forced to use tools centered on artificial intelligence algorithms that can help us better predict the very same things that screening programs are designed to do. Either way, these unintended consequences of screening programs are worth paying attention to.

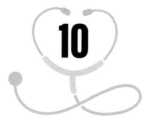

Ghost in the Machine

The real problem is not whether machines think but whether men do.

—B. F. Skinner

That artificial intelligence is interwoven with health care in the twenty-first century is undeniable. The only question left to answer is, How much more reliant are we going to become as we strive to solve some of our most vexing health care problems?

To think about the power of artificial intelligence today, here are some examples of applications of artificial intelligence in health care that you are all eminently familiar with, even though you may not know it: Using technology to "crawl" social media to see what patients and doctors are saying about your drug to better understand aspects of pharmacovigilance. Using artificial intelligence as a bench researcher interested in a new pathway for drug development but unsure as to the current peer-reviewed literature in that space. Or a market access/reimbursement team looks for relevant reference cases from the National Institute for

Health and Care Excellence to make cost-effectiveness arguments with a payer by using artificial intelligence to model budget impact and therapy uptake within a defined population. Some
simpler methods to achieve these goals are to replace outdated
keyword searches or some hybrid keyword-semantic model with
a 100 percent semantic model. In *Google Semantic Search*, author David Amerland concludes that semantic search is a game
changer.[1] If this sounds familiar, it is because Google (and others)
has incorporated this into their search algorithm under the Hum-
mingbird project moniker. The underlying foundation of Google
and all the other semantic search companies is knowledge graphs.[2]
The simple idea behind knowledge graphs is that each subject of
interest is represented by a node, and these nodes form connections with other nodes (sometimes referred to as parent-child relationships) and the connections between these nodes grow stronger
and stronger as the algorithm incorporates and internalizes more
user data. The beauty of semantic search platforms is that the
knowledge graphs are individualized based on the user's nodal
strength. If I search for information related to diabetes, soon the
semantic search platform will understand that I am interested in
information on diabetes and will dynamically continue to popu-
late my dashboard with anything and everything diabetes related. Diabetic retinopathy. Diabetic neuropathy. Diabetic foot
ulcers. Diabetic hand syndrome. Patient information on diabetes.
Clinical trial information on diabetes. News about diabetes. Social media chatter about diabetes medications. You do not need
to keep going back and querying the term *diabetes* any longer.

But the value of artificial intelligence in health care goes way
beyond the ability to better contextualize search queries and return more relevant results, doesn't it? I mean, getting back 570
million search results in less than a second on the search query
term *diabetes* is infinitely less important than getting back five
hundred meaningful search results in three seconds. Or ten

seconds. The time difference is literally a few blinks of the eye. Almost anyone, including patients who are searching for important information on disease management, is willing to trade off a few seconds for more meaningful data. The less data you have to sift through, the faster you can make decisions. In health care, whether it's drug discovery or disease diagnosis, speed matters. The irony should not be lost on the reader: by taking more time, we save time. Now there's a novelty.

The power of artificial intelligence has vast application beyond better contextualization of searches. Consider the big data dilemma in life sciences, which has received an incredible amount of attention over the past few years. The dilemma is this: with ever-growing and vast amounts of data becoming available to us, how do we harness this information to, among other things, better diagnose disease, deliver health care, differentiate between why some patients respond to a drug and others do not, listen to the voice of the patient as they describe side effects, and enhance drug discovery.

Well, a few of the behemoth companies, such as Google, Amazon, and Apple, are working feverishly to wrangle large amounts of data to address some (not all) of these problems. Not the consumer-facing problems that receive all the attention (wearable health devices) but the problems that address the frustration of providing relevance, contextualization, and uncovering meaningful patterns with the mountains of health data out there. Then there are other companies that, by virtue of their lack of scale and size—and the natural media attention that comes along with scale and size—are quietly making giant leaps in this field. This is not to suggest that wearables do not provide redeeming value, cannot solve some of our health care problems, and do not have a place in the conversation. But we are not there yet with wearables. There are obvious technological problems related to functionality. There are access problems related to cost and the exclusion of vast swaths of the global population who simply cannot afford these devices. There are the ever-present privacy concerns with technology that accesses your sensitive health data and stores it in the cloud. But the barrier to wide adoption of wearables also centers on a more rudimentary problem: changing behavior. It is one thing to measure the number of steps we take in a day or one's cardiac enzymes, blood sugar levels, and any other number of clinically relevant lab parameters, but it is another thing to change the patient's behavior with this information. The gap between recording health information and using that information to galvanize behavior change is colossal. So, let's leave wearables out of the discussion for the time being.

To return to the issue of big data, the answer to the data dilemma lies in a subset of artificial intelligence known as machine learning. Machine learning is the name given to output derived from algorithms that use statistics to find patterns in massive (or less-than-massive) amounts of data without having been explicitly programmed to do so. Data, by definition, can include lab values, words in a Subjective Objective Assessment Plan (SOAP) note, MRI images, X-rays, adverse effects articulated by patients, you name it. If it can be digitally stored, it can be fed into a machine-learning algorithm. Machine learning is the secret sauce that powers many of the household products that we routinely use every day: recommendation systems such as those on Netflix, YouTube, and Spotify; search engines such as Google and Baidu; social-media feeds such as Facebook and Twitter; voice assistants such as Siri and Alexa. The list goes on.[3] As Karen Hao states in her primer on machine learning from *MIT Technology Review*, "in all of these instances, each platform is collecting as much data about you as possible—what genres you like watching, what links you are clicking, which statuses you are reacting to—and using machine learning to make a highly educated guess about what you might want next. Or, in the case of a voice assistant, about which words match best with the funny sounds coming out of your mouth."[4]

Related to machine learning and the notion of using statistics and data to find patterns in almost anything, is its close cousin known as deep learning. Deep learning uses a technique called deep neural networks to enhance a machine's ability to find even the smallest patterns between variables in a data set.[5] Think of machine learning like the microscope you got for your eighth birthday. It cost $19.99, and it worked. You could see stuff through the lens. Now think of deep learning as the $30,000 medical grade microscope you worked with when you were in a major academic hospital with all the big budgets for capital equipment purchases.

As Hao states in her article, three main branches of machine (or deep) learning fundamentally guide our understanding of this discipline. The first is known as *supervised learning*. In this branch of machine learning, we basically label all the data we eventually intend to feed into the machine so that the machine knows what patterns to look for. Think of this as us telling the machine that the labels in a data set are "increased thirst" and "frequent urination." And then us asking the machine to figure out the diagnosis (the well-informed readers out there will forgive the rudimentary example). The machine will start to piece together that the inherent pattern gluing the data points together in this fictitious example with the labels that we have provided is that all these patients have diabetes. Or you can think of this like I do: a trail of breadcrumbs that leads the machine to where it needs to go. The second branch is known as *unsupervised learning*. In unsupervised learning, data have no labels. The machine just looks for whatever patterns it can find. To follow our earlier example, we give the machine no breadcrumbs. We take it out into the middle of the woods, à la Hansel and Gretel, and see whether it can find its way home. There are no labels provided. The machine tells *us* what it sees. The third branch that Hao describes is *reinforcement learning*. In this last branch of machine learning, "the reinforcement algorithm learns by trial and error to achieve a clear objective. It tries out lots of different things and is rewarded or penalized depending on whether its behaviors help or hinder it from reaching its objective."[6]

With these facts in hand, the motivation for machine learning to address issues such as accelerating drug discovery, lowering its cost, and identifying lead candidates for drug trials holds tremendous promise. Think about a use case as follows: the pharmaceutical industry faces many headwinds as we enter the third decade of this century—the greatest of which may be the continual loss of branded medications due to expiring patents. As companies face this patent cliff, pressure increases to develop drugs faster and cheaper to continue to replace products that contribute to top-line revenue. Drug development can cost from $650 million to $2.6 billion and take anywhere from five years to twenty years.[7] Today's big pharmaceutical companies recognize that they do not have the human capital, financial capital, or time to deploy against this issue in a meaningful way. They have collectively heard a lot about machine learning, and their own data scientists are itching to form a partnership.

But before diving in headfirst, we must acknowledge that in today's world of machine learning, three fundamental blind spots should be addressed.

First, many of today's machine learning algorithms are designed for simple, linear tasks. In a linear system, the relationship between the input and the output are proportional and rather easy to predict. If you smoke ten packs of cigarettes per day, you will likely suffer from emphysema, or COPD, or some other respiratory illness. But the world is full of nonlinear complexity. In these systems, no proportionality and no simple causality exist between the magnitude of responses and the strength of their stimuli: small changes can have striking and unanticipated effects, whereas large stimuli will not always lead to drastic changes in a system's behavior.[8] Nonlinear systems often appear to be chaotic, unpredictable, or counterintuitive and solving them holds tremendous application. To further illustrate this point, in mathematics and physical sciences, a nonlinear system is a system in which the change of the output is not proportional to the change of the input. For example, the stock market, weather patterns, or disease. A single word from the chair of the Federal Reserve about fiscal policy can send the stock market into a spiral or skyrocketing upward. A half-degree temperature change somewhere on the planet can have immeasurable effect for centuries to come. A single mutation, inversion, or translation of a gene can result in devastating effects for human health. These are all examples of nonlinear complexity—the scenario in which a lack of proportionality exists between the exposure and the outcome. And all exemplify the reason machine learning methods need to be able to solve for this problem.

A second challenge with today's machine learning methods is that many of them are dependent on big data. In a different time, place, and context, perhaps a lot of data is not a bad thing. It is, in some regards, even desirable. The more data points we have, the higher our degree of certainty and confidence about the patterns that we see in those data points. But the cost and time involved with aggregating huge volumes of data and then cleaning the data of variables that may interfere with interpretation are not insignificant and may delay attempts at resolving some of our more pressing health care problems, such as the optimization of clinical trials to better understand patient nonresponse or the discovery of lead drug candidates to advance into clinical trials. However, some platforms can learn from as few as a couple of hundred data points, with equivalent or superior insights to traditional big data machine learning predictive models, and help us reduce failures significantly across many of our most pressing problem areas in health care. These solutions uniquely predict the root cause for failure across the drug development cycle, including identification of specific patient subpopulations and placebo response (or lack thereof). While we may be cynical of the need to wring our hands about this because the poor, ol' pharmaceutical industry needs help to develop drugs so that they continue to make reams and reams of money, remember this: someone has to pay for this technology (the public sector is likely not a good candidate), and the adoption of this technology at scale allows for the hospital researchers and other public sector scientists, who do not have the pharmaceutical company budgets, to benefit (albeit down the road) from this innovation.

Finally, the issue of opacity is a troubling problem with some machine learning platforms. Known as black box syndrome, explainability or interpretability, this problem is exacerbated in industries such as health care, which are heavily regulated and where submitting a drug for regulatory approval requires a precise ability to show how a drug acts in a particular way to affect a particular disease pathway. It is the ability to understand what the system is doing and the basis for its recommendations that proves to be crucial. As Eric Bender describes in his *Undark* article "Unpacking the Black Box in Artificial Intelligence for Medicine," "in a 2019 retrospective study of mammograms from about 40,000 women at Massachusetts General Hospital, the researchers found the deep learning system substantially outperformed the current gold-standard approach on a test set of about 4,000 of these women." Bender goes on to state that, with further testing and validation, this deep learning system may become part of routine care at the hospital.[9] Herein lies an important nugget of information about deep learning that I have not touched on yet. I have focused on cost, time, and efficiency as the raison d'être for machine learning. What about accuracy? What about the fact that the machine is potentially simply better than we are as a species at whatever we ask the machine to do? In health care, this has profound implications.

Regina Barzilay, a computer scientist from the Massachusetts Institute of Technology, who developed this deep learning program for Massachusetts General Hospital, is described by Bender as confident that we can truly understand deep learning systems. Further, she argues that we currently use other types of machine learning that are equally unexplainable and we do not seem bothered by it in the least. She opines that "medicine is crammed with advanced technologies that work in ways that clinicians really don't understand—for instance, the magnetic resonance imaging (MRI) that gathers the mammography data to begin with."[10] She may have a point.

Last year a team at Google used data on eye scans from over one hundred twenty-five thousand patients to build an algorithm that could detect retinopathy, the number one cause of blindness in some parts of the world, with over 90 percent accuracy, on par with board-certified ophthalmologists. These results had constraints; humans could not always fully comprehend why the models made the decisions they made. Other such examples are also readily available. To be truthful, some resist these methods, calling for a complete ban on using non-explainable algorithms in high-impact areas such as health because they may lead to forced, faulty, or unethical logic. Earlier this year, France's minister of state for the digital sector flatly stated that any algorithm that cannot be explained should not be used. The naysayers are, indeed, loud. A group of clinicians wrote in the *British Medical Journal* that

> many popular machine learning algorithms are essentially black boxes—oracular inference engines that render verdicts without any accompanying justification. This problem has become especially pressing with passage of the European Union's latest General Data Protection Regulation (GDPR), which some scholars argue provides citizens with a "right to explanation." Now, any institution engaged in algorithmic decision making is legally required to justify those decisions to any person whose data they hold on request, a challenge that most are ill equipped to meet.[11]

Essentially, this amounts to a grandfather clause argument. Forget about what came before machine learning and that we may not understand why the phacoemulsification machine for cataract surgery recommends a certain setting or the therapy unit we use to treat diabetic foot wounds asks us to engage certain levels of negative pressure to form granulation tissue at the site of the wound. Heck, let's even forget about the fact that we do not really know how medical cannabis should be dosed for the optimal management of chronic pain, insomnia, post-traumatic stress disorder, and other ailments, but we continue to dose it anyway. Let's forget about all this. The point is that there is a lot in medicine that we cannot explain. It seems, however, the argument is that those other technologies and therapeutics are in wide adoption and utilization and, therefore, they get a pass on the lack of explainability. They have been grandfathered in.

So, there you have it. A promising technology, like many others before it, that has friction points that may prevent wider adoption. This is not the first time we have seen this, and it will not be the last. But, as with all other such examples through the course of history, knowing what the pitfalls are and having our eyes wide open, will help us unleash the true power of machine learning in health care in the years to come. But adopting and unleashing new technology is not only about learning from the past and keeping our eyes open. It's about understanding that we will have expectations about new technologies and face realities about new technologies. How we close the gap between the expectations and realities might be the key.

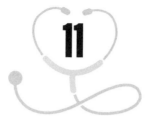

The Eye of the Storm

Remember that the storm is a good opportunity for the pine and the cypress to show their strength and their stability.　　　　　　—HO CHI MINH

The way people respond to tornado warnings may have public health implications.

In Michael Lewis's book *The Fifth Risk*, the author describes the complete chaos and apathy as it related to transitioning from the Obama administration to the Trump administration and more specifically the complete lack of direction on important policy issues. In particular, the reader is taken into the world of NOAA (National Oceanic and Atmospheric Administration) and how its raison d'être was completely abandoned by the Trump administration, its funding stripped, and its policy directives ignored. NOAA is largely responsible for understanding and predicting weather and climate changes and sharing that information with the public. That the Trump administration stripped NOAA of much-needed funding should come as no surprise to anyone, given the administration's disdain for anything that remotely positions climate change as a tangible manifestation rooted in man-made etiology.

However, what is eminently interesting is a section near the end of the book in which some of the administrators of this large and incredibly important part of the American government grapple with a seemingly innocuous question: Why do people, when faced with advanced warning of imminent tornado threats, refuse to take heed and simply stay put? In an interesting twist, the department hired a bunch of behavioral scientists to help them answer this question. One conclusion of this research was that "normal humans don't understand probabilities and cannot translate wind speed or rain rate into tangible worries."[1] Simply put, people want to know what this high wind or biblical amount of rain *is going to do to their house*. Not what it is going to do to every (other) house. They do not need the scientific jargon. They need specificity, not large generalizations.

As interesting an observation as this is, it is incomplete. I know you find this obvious. Many, including me, have advocated and warned about the perils of health illiteracy and the need to speak to patients in a language that they comprehend and that allows them to make informed decisions. The same is true of overall public policy illiteracy—it is not just a health literacy thing. But perhaps the most interesting behavioral insight from NOAA's work comes not from the fact that we need to eliminate the nuances of scientific jargon when we communicate public policy directives to the population at large but in the way individuals internalize risk, uncertainty, and their own personal invincibility. What NOAA researchers set out to uncover was how and when complacency turned into urgency. Why do some people ignore a tornado warning when given days of notice while others pack up everything they have, throw it into a car, and head for the highway?

This behavior has important implications for health care. Because we know people ignore health warnings also, while others will modify their behavior in light of the same warnings.

What NOAA researchers found was incredibly startling. It is not that people were ignoring the tornado warnings that the National Weather Service was sending out or that they had not heard the warnings. These people were aware of the warnings. They watched television, read the papers, tuned into newstalk radio, and conversed with their neighbors. They just thought the tornado would never hit *them*. They thought this way because a tornado had never hit them before even though they had heard the same warnings for years and years. Why does this happen?

Part of the answer may lie in what is known as the *optimism bias*. Tali Sharot explains it as follows in a 2011 paper: "The optimism bias is defined as the difference between a person's expectation and the outcome that follows. If expectations are better than reality, the bias is optimistic; if reality is better than expected, the bias is pessimistic. The extent of the optimism bias is thus measured empirically by recording an individual's expectations before an event unfolds and contrasting those with the outcomes that transpire."[2] To be straightforward about the whole thing, people who ignore tornado warnings and health warnings have a very high optimism bias. They simply do not think they are going to get cancer, a heart attack, or have a tornado blow the roof off their house. Sharot explains some of the underlying mechanisms about the optimism bias that were elucidated from research in her lab. Essentially her group found that an optimism bias is maintained in the face of contrary or disconfirming evidence because people update their beliefs more in response to positive information about the future than to negative information about the future. Sharot illustrates the example using scenarios involving burglary and Alzheimer's disease to demonstrate the point. People are first asked to estimate the chances of being robbed or being afflicted by Alzheimer's disease in their lifetime. Then Sharot's research team provided study participants with the average frequencies of these events occurring in the general population. Then, participants were asked to update their estimates of these events occurring to them after having been made aware of the population average. Unsurprisingly, in situations where study participants had underestimated the likelihood of an event occurring in their lives (i.e., they think that their chances of being afflicted with Alzheimer's is 20% but the data show that it is 40 percent in the general population), they did not update their estimate much. However, when shown data that depicted an overestimation of the event occurring in their lives (i.e., they think that their chances of being afflicted with Alzheimer's is 40% but the data shows that it is 20% in the general population), they substantially modified their estimate to more closely match the population average.[3]

For those who are wondering about the biology behind this, Sharot explains that this selective updating of estimates when individuals are presented with discordant information between expectations and reality of events is mediated by the frontal lobe of our brain. Essentially, she points out, "when optimistic individuals are confronted with unexpected statistics about the likelihood of encountering negative events, their right inferior frontal gyrus exhibits reduced coding of information that calls for a negative update."[4] In essence, the brain of optimistic people ignores what it is being told and, like computer software, simply does not update itself in the face of this information with a new (and more accurate) expectation.

And we do not really need to use burglary and Alzheimer's examples. Think about the COVID-19 pandemic. Yes, COVID-19 is a multifaceted issue and the behavior of a single individual (or a population) cannot be explained by a single factor. But isn't this optimism bias, in part, exactly what is happening? Are we not witnessing a series of individual optimistic biases that morph into data points right before our very eyes? Are there not millions of people around the world who *do not* think that they are going to contract COVID-19 or die from COVID-19 despite the epidemiological data that we now have in our possession? Of course, this is not the only factor at play, but the idea that people, faced with cognitively dissonant population averages from their own expectations about personal disease susceptibility, are more or less likely to adjust their behavior, depending on their starting point, has stark implications for the spread of the disease. And as Sharot pointed out in one of her examples she used in a TED Talk, we are, at times, faced with a statistical conundrum when dealing with optimism biases. Actually, a statistical impossibility. If you ask people how likely they are to contract COVID-19 relative to the rest of the population and to rank themselves from the bottom quartile (most likely to contract COVID-19) to the highest quartile (least likely to contract COVID-19), the vast majority of people will probably cluster in the highest quartile. Now, think about this for a moment. This means that most of us think we are less likely than the next person to contract COVID-19. But it is simply not possible that this belief can hold true in actuality for COVID-19. Or cancer. Or Alzheimer's. And it is not a complicated leap to see why this bias has such a profound impact with respect to COVID-19. I mean, the disease was able to spread at an approximate rate of every infected person transmitting the disease to two or three other people (known as the R_0 number). So, if most people are optimistic about their chances of *not* getting COVID-19, then how exactly did they get it.

The fundamental point about the optimism bias and the misaligned expectations between what you expect to happen and the reality of what actually happens that we do not really address is, What happens when the bias is wrong? What happens when people tell you that they estimate their chances of contracting COVID-19 is less than 1 percent and you tell them that the data shows the chances are closer to 5 percent based on diagnostic testing and they get the illness. Do they change their future behavior? Does the right inferior frontal gyrus now enhance the coding of information that calls for a negative update?

The phenomenon of optimism bias is implicated in other important areas of health care and is not only a problem related to real-world patients. There is some research that suggests this may be a problem in clinical trial patients as well. Chalmers and colleagues report that

> optimism bias has several serious implications. One is the creation of unrealistic expectations, for both patients and clinicians, of the likely benefits of new treatments in randomised trials. For example, in the early 1990s, clinicians participating in a trial of a new radiotherapy treatment for head and neck cancer were asked for their expectations of the likely outcome. Their responses revealed a high level of optimism, the consensus being that the new treatment would reduce mortality by around 30%. In the event, the trial found no evidence that the new treatment was an advance. Furthermore, an analysis based on a cohort of 57 radiotherapy trials done between 1968 and 2002 and involving nearly 13 000 patients has shown that innovative treatments are as likely to be inferior to established treatments as they are to be superior.[5]

What does this all mean in practical terms? For one thing, that the misalignment between expectations and reality with respect to experimental or unapproved drugs may inadvertently drive recruitment into clinical trials by overly optimistic clinicians and patients who might assign an unrealistic expectation of efficacy or symptom management and control toward these therapies. Undoubtedly, there may be other potential issues, but this one is the most salient.

Finally, there is another meaningful area on the health care spectrum where an optimism bias may be problematic. Ahn et al. looked at patients' optimism bias in the context of responses to risk disclosures in direct-to-consumer prescription drug advertising, and their results are illuminating. The researchers surveyed just over four hundred people and found that "consumers who show a tendency to believe that they are at less risk of experiencing adverse reactions to prescription drugs than their peers are less likely to pay attention to the risk disclosure or intend to seek further information about the health risks of drugs."[6] There are obvious methodological problems with many studies. No study is perfect, and some are less perfect than others. This is one of those studies. It is a survey; the sample was recruited through a market research firm, and the overwhelming majority of respondents (92.3%) were white, which makes generalizability a challenge. The directional results of this research are potentially important. What this research portends is that people who have a lower optimism bias about their own likelihood of experiencing side effects of prescription drugs are "more likely to pay attention to risk disclosures, more likely to perceive that the risk disclosures are important to them, and more likely to show intentions to seek further risk information through alternative sources than those with a high optimistic bias about the likelihood of experiencing side-effects of prescription drugs."[7] The problem, as you have all undoubtedly recognized, is that we need proper studies that allow us to truly establish a causal link or a strong association between these variables of optimism bias, risk disclosure, and outcomes. Even then, if we are able to establish a meaningful relationship, the question is how we modify risk disclosure communication to different groups of people to mitigate the problem.

Surely, you all see the health care corollaries in clinical trials, in everyday patients, and in how we communicate risk disclosure for prescription drugs. Do clinicians and public health officials know the importance of this inherent optimism bias and how it may affect health behavior? Well, according to Sharot, one group of clinicians probably knows more about it than anyone else: psychologists and psychiatrists because at least one group of humans fail to show positively biased expectations. That group comprises individuals suffering from depression.[8] Other researchers have shown that while nondepressed humans expect the future to be slightly better than reality, individuals with *mild* depression show no bias when predicting future events, and people with *severe* depression tend to expect things to be worse than they turn out. [9] Therefore, while optimistic biases are common in the majority of nondepressed people, there is no such manifestation with depressed individuals. As Strunk et al. point out, pessimism is actually one of the hallmark symptoms of depression, according to *The Diagnostic and Statistical Manual of Mental Disorders (DSM IV)*.[10]

But the optimism bias does not and cannot explain everything about people who ignore tornado warnings and public health advice. The other synchronous interpretation from this example is that those who do not listen to their doctors and to public health officials (and there are large numbers of them) have an invincibility complex that the tornado cynics also possess. This is quite different than being optimistic about something not happening. The optimism bias is, at its core, a misalignment between the expectations of an event and its ultimate reality. An invincibility complex is more like an individual knowing that an event can occur with no misalignment between what is expected and what happens. It is simply a belief that the individual will not be affected. I know there is an 80 percent chance of a tornado hitting my house and that is pretty much what I expect to happen. But I will be all right even if it does happen. Researchers have studied this invincibility complex in a health care setting before, and, to no surprise, there is a strong association between it, the acceptance of health promotion messages, and age.[11] Younger people are more likely to shrug off potential health concerns and preventative public health messages or guidance from their clinician than older people are. This is true of drunk driving and sexually transmitted diseases ("it won't happen to me") and, as elucidated earlier, a marked problem in the context of COVID-19, where the infection and fatality rates for those under the age of thirty are quite low, but the risk of transmitting the disease to more susceptible populations is high. While the goal of this chapter is not necessarily to introduce solutions, evidence supports the involvement of the target audience in shaping and planning health promotions to their peers.[12]

The larger extensions to health care are downright scary. The idea that people do not need to exercise, to get enough sleep, to eat a balanced diet high in fruits and vegetables and low in red meat, or to quit smoking and reduce salt intake and alcohol consumption. This notion that people will not get heart disease or diabetes or cancer or some other disease. It will not happen to them because it has never happened to them before. They have always been healthy. They are invincible. As Michael Lewis recounts in his book, many things *can* happen to you. But only a tiny subset of all those things actually *do* happen. It is that critical subset of experiences that shapes your worldview and determines your risk, uncertainty, and invincibility profile.[13]

Want proof? Ask people who have established heart disease, a cancer in remission, or some other similar ailment whether they are more careful and attentive about listening to the doctor's advice once they have already been sick. Want more proof? Ask someone who has been through a tornado whether they will ever ignore another warning again. We do not want people to get a disease or an illness just for the sake of having some experience with disease and illness so that their optimism threshold has been lowered or their invincibility bias has been shattered. This is not desirable. We would prefer a completely healthy society of course. This is not possible.

In-between these two extremes lies an important lesson. This lesson that balances these two extremes of invincibility and optimism offset against disease and illness is magnificently illustrated in how we have chosen to try to get back to "normal" health care during the COVID-19 pandemic.

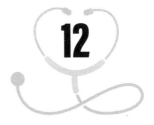

12

Homesick

> Everything will be alright in the end; and if it is not alright, then it is not yet the end. —DEBORAH MOGGACH, *The Best Exotic Marigold Hotel*

As counterintuitive as it might sound, you might be risking your health by not risking your health.

In the new world order that was forced on us as a result of COVID-19, a slew of behavioral health nudges emanated from hundreds of countries around the world that were a matter of life and death as the pandemic continued to wreak havoc around the world. Chief among those nudges was the holy triad of quarantine, shelter-in-place, and stay-at-home. Take your pick, really. They all had the same basic intent and end goal: do not go out and needlessly expose yourself or others to the virus. Unless you were a frontline worker, you needed to stay at home as much as possible. We had to flatten the curve and the R_0 (pronounced R naught), otherwise known as the reproduction number, from spiraling out of control. In the absence of a vaccine or larger population-level herd immunity, we needed that R_0 to be below 1, or, at the very least, at 1 if we had any chance of tamping down the spread of COVID-19.[1]

As we stared at the numbers of infected and dead scroll across our television screens on a nightly basis, we realized that there was a massive health care implication, outside of the obvious direct impact of COVID-19, that came with these stay-at-home nudges: *people were afraid to leave their house.* And with good reason. The disease was still active, was incredibly infectious, and had a devastating effect on the most vulnerable in society, such as the elderly and immunocompromised.

But we are setting ourselves up for a devastating reckoning. For it is one thing to reduce the number of visits to your local grocery store from three times per week to once a week or to refrain from going to the bank every day and, instead, use online or electronic banking to pay your bills and transfer money. But people are skipping much-needed medical appointments. Yes, telehealth interventions have helped (more on that later) but only to the extent that individuals have access to the technology to make this happen. By individuals, I mean both patients and clinicians. Let us be honest, it is not just a question of access to technology but the nature of the disease or illness that lends itself to management through broadband that matters. Some illnesses require an in-person visit to ensure proper delivery of care and follow-on testing and monitoring. The degree to which the government enables clinicians to bill for services rendered through telehealth platforms by reducing the legislation and red tape involved is a major factor in this equation, too. People are postponing again previously canceled elective procedures that had been rescheduled. Think about the mind-bending gymnastics involved in that sentence. COVID-19 forced the cancellation of relatively routine hip, knee, cataract, cardiovascular, and other surgical procedures (some readers will rightly argue that no surgical procedure is routine) as hospitals around the world sought to both prepare for the mass influx of COVID-19 patients and protect the vulnerable from unnecessary exposure to the virus. Although we may not lump them in with traditional chronic disease management, the complete abandonment of dental and eye care should not go unnoticed, as well as higher-risk procedures such as cancer and solid organ transplant surgeries. The effect of delayed cancer care is highlighted by Jones et al., who report in *The Lancet* that "management and follow-up of patients with cancer is also affected by the COVID-19 pandemic. Many patients with cancer, especially those undergoing chemotherapy, radical radiotherapy, and immunotherapy, are at greater risk from the symptoms and sequelae of COVID-19."[2] The authors also state that "screening, case identification, and the referral in symptomatic cancer diagnosis have all been affected by the COVID-19 pandemic. UK national cancer screening programmes—accounting for approximately 5% of all cancer diagnoses each year—have been suspended. Consequently, early diagnoses from screening will be delayed and symptom-based diagnosis of cancer will become more important."[3] And this is probably true of almost every nation in the Organisation for Economic Co-operation and Development regarding cancer care management, screening, and referral. There is no reason to believe that the United Kingdom's approach is any different than its OECD cousins.

As some countries emerged from the depths of this pandemic, hospitals and individual and group practices began to call patients back in for those procedures, assessments, and disease management interventions only to be met with resistance. Or maybe fear is a more accurate word in some respects. In other situations, apathy might be a more appropriate word.

Perhaps most troubling, which foreshadows greater calamity, is that families did not vaccinate their children as the Centers for Disease Control and Prevention and the World Health Organization had warned.[4] The *New York Times* reported in 2020 that "in a new study released by the Centers for Disease Control and Prevention, the vaccination rates in May for children under 2 years old in Michigan fell to alarming rates, including fewer than half of infants 5 months or younger."[5] The CDC and WHO's prediction actually happened (figure 17).

In the United States, children are vaccinated against hepatitis B, whooping cough, rotavirus, diphtheria, tetanus, measles, polio,

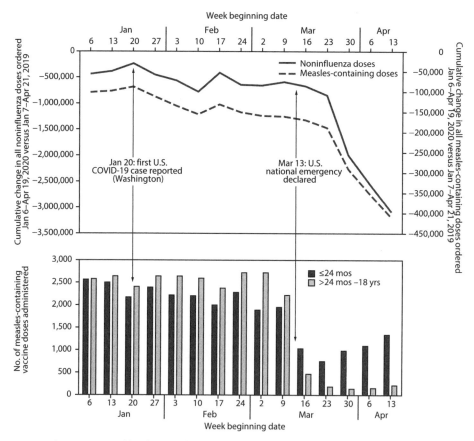

Figure 17. Weekly changes in Vaccines for Children Program (VFC) provider orders and Vaccine Safety Datalink (VSD) doses administered for routine pediatric vaccines—United States, January 6–April 19, 2020. Centers for Disease Control and Prevention.

and chicken pox, among other diseases according to a recent *Vox* article. The author reminds us that researchers have estimated that for every year children receive all the recommended childhood immunizations, some twenty million illnesses and forty thousand deaths are prevented.[6] Lest we think that this is a first-world problem, public health experts have warned that approximately one hundred million children could be at risk for measles because no less than twenty-four low- to middle-income countries are pausing or postponing their national immunization programs, including Bolivia, Chad, Chile, Colombia, Djibouti, the Dominican Republic, Ethiopia, Honduras, Lebanon, Nepal, Paraguay, Somalia, South Sudan, and Uzbekistan.[7] The countries least prepared to deal with a global pandemic of a novel virus that has the potential to overwhelm their health care systems are potentially facing an onslaught from a disease for which the R_o is 12–18, which means that each person with measles would, on average, infect twelve to eighteen other people in a totally susceptible population.[8] For these nations, the public health challenges are staggering.

In-home visits by physical, rehabilitation, and occupational therapists were severely curtailed with no visible revival of those crucial health care services. As new and renewal prescriptions were delivered by contactless method, the important role of the pharmacist in educating and counseling patients about medication adherence and the management of adverse events had disappeared. Then, of course, there was and continues to be the mental health impact of COVID-19: anxiety, worry, and stress about exacerbating preexisting conditions or avoiding medical care due to fear of exposure, causing needless morbidity, pain, and increased mortality. The psychological toll of this pandemic on the non-COVID-19 patient is yet to be completely elucidated, but it is sure to reveal itself over the months and years to come.

There you have it. From the dentist to the physical therapist to the surgeon and everyone in-between, the non-COVID-19 landscape of health care has come to a grinding halt as people simply venture anywhere but near a health care facility. The cataclysmic manifestation of this problem, while sure to be diffuse, may lie most noticeably in the effects that we see with respect to chronic disease management. The diabetic and hypertensive patients who are skipping checkups and routine follow-up visits because the mortality profile of COVID-19 suggests that one of the groups most susceptible has underlying comorbidities such as metabolic syndrome and cardiovascular disease. Of course, the respiratory patients—those with chronic obstructive pulmonary disease, bronchitis, and asthma—are in the same boat as the diabetics and hypertensives. The impact of this disease on the lungs is well documented. And then we have a whole other group—psoriasis patients and rheumatoid arthritis patients and Crohn's disease patients and dialysis patients.

And there is some evidence, albeit small, that points to the potential for a real problem in the months and years that follow our ability to control COVID-19. A study published following the 2002–2004 SARS outbreak showed that chronic-care hospitalizations for diabetes dropped precipitously during the crisis but rebounded afterward and, to no surprise, public health and health policy experts are worried that similar problems could crop up as a result of the COVID-19 pandemic.[9]

This tsunami of chronic disease management patients who are missing regular and routine care, the reticence to rebook previously canceled elective surgeries, and the alarming reductions in important childhood vaccinations are all exacerbated by multiple factors. First, the COVID-19 vaccine strategy, which included development, testing, and distribution, was hideously inefficient and riddled with confusion, delays, and uncertainty. We have learned that the process of getting from lab to pharmacy shelf is teeming with unforeseen complexities. Second, the widespread agreement that there is going to be a potentially calamitous return of this virus in the colder months in Northern Hemisphere countries each and every year bodes ill for us. But there is another factor that may prevent non-COVID-19 patients from getting back to routine care in the foreseeable future and that is the utter economic devastation that this pandemic is having on the health care system—to speak nothing of the utter devastation it is having on households' ability to pay for the care they seek.

Some hospitals and doctors may no longer be there when patients try to come back. Call it early retirement, bankruptcy, or a new operating model. Call it whatever you want. The impact on patient care is the same. Fewer doctors seeing the same number of patients with the same diseases.

As reported by CNBC, "because many hospitals cancelled or delayed elective procedures to make space for a potential flood of COVID-19 patients they were losing millions of dollars per day just staying open. In April of 2020, the American Hospital Association estimated that hospitals were bleeding more than $50 billion per month."[10] Dr. Bob Wachter, chair of the Department of Medicine at University of California, San Francisco, is quoted in the same article, reminding us that many hospitals survive on razor-thin margins to begin with, which are, in large part, manageable because (high margin) patients with employer-based or private insurance offset the lower-margin Medicare and Medicaid patients: "Since hospitals, with some notable exceptions, are paid based on the number of procedures they perform whether that's a surgery or an X-ray at their imaging center, they make money on some patients and lose money on others."[11]

And Richard Pollack, CEO of the American Hospital Association, which represents five thousand hospitals, health care systems, networks, and other providers of care (about forty-three thousand individual members) lays it squarely on the line: "We're being faced with what I would call a triple whammy. We have the increased expenses that have been incurred in terms of preparing for the surge and caring for the COVID-19 patients. And then we have the decreased revenues associated with having shut down regular operations in terms of scheduled procedures. You combine that with the increased number of uninsured as a result of the economic situation, and you've got a triple whammy there."[12] As we have learned about how to operate our hospitals in the face of this pandemic, this bleak outlook recedes further into memory, but it is, nevertheless, something to be mindful of since no hospital can run itself without patients. Even though we have learned a ton as policy makers, epidemiologists, and health care providers, the reality is that we need patients to have learned just as much.

As promised, we will now examine the role of telemedicine solutions. This is where these platforms expose an undeniable economic and practical issue. Yes, telemedicine allows some patients some of the time to manage their disease without interruption or exacerbation of their condition. Hospitals are not averse to using these platforms as demonstrated by the staggering increase in virtual visits implemented by Ochsner Health in New Orleans, where they have completed more than one hundred twenty thousand virtual visits during the pandemic times of 2020 compared to a lowly thirty-three hundred in all of 2019.[13] That is the good news. The flip side is that telemedicine does not provide nearly the same revenue streams to hospitals as in-patient visits do. As Dr. Wachter opines, "treating a patient in person also lets hospitals collect facility and technical fees, and possibly add procedures that can't be done remotely, like a lab test or an X-ray."[14] Furthermore, the data from large hospital systems that have immense budgets and the resources to stagger their way through this crisis belie the reality facing the small individual health care practitioner who has seen patient volume evaporate: the economic impact of COVID-19 may figuratively kill the primary care and specialty practices of thousands of US physicians. As Oliver Brooks, MD, and president of the National Medical Association said in a recent article, these practices "don't have large cash reserves in which they can wait three months to get money coming from the federal government."[15] All of these sobering numbers make the effect of COVID-19 on health care more far-reaching than previously considered. Some, though, like James Robinson, professor of health economics at the University of California, Berkeley, are envisioning a potential silver lining from the anticipated extinction of many small solo practices: consolidation. With increasing frequency, we have seen independent practices amalgamated into larger health delivery systems through mergers and buyouts. Robinson believes this, too, will occur with COVID-19.[16] And the evidence is mixed on the long-term implications of this. There is evidence that shows amalgamation and consolidation within health care can "lead to better communication between doctors, more efficient use of testing and scans, and more cost-effective treatment."[17] The equally compelling evidence is that this is not the case, with some peer-reviewed data showing that hospital mergers, consolidation, amalgamation, and physician buyouts have increased insurance prices for patients. In areas with high hospital consolidation and high proportions of hospital-owned physician practices, health insurance premiums cost up to 12 percent more than in areas with average levels of consolidation.[18]

What about the private health insurance marketplace and its impact on this topic? David Cutler, the Otto Eckstein Professor of Applied Economics in the Department of Economics at Harvard University, with secondary appointments at the Kennedy School of Government and the School of Public Health, reminds us that "historically, health care has been relatively immune from recessions. People get sick during both good and bad times, so demand for medical care is relatively constant across the business cycle. Furthermore, health insurance reduces the out-of-pocket costs for care that people face; thus, many sick people—at least those with health insurance—can still afford to visit physicians."[19] But he goes on to opine that today's private insurance is vastly different than it used to be even a decade ago with 25 percent of people who have private insurance facing a deductible of $2,000 or more. This level of exposure to high deductible care is, as Cutler says, more than four times what it was in 2010.[20] The natural outgrowth of this reality is that even patients who have employer-based or private insurance are taciturn about seeking much-needed care. While it may have little to do with fear of contracting the virus, the result is the same. Delayed diagnosis, care, and treatment will exacerbate preexisting conditions and new illnesses, resulting in another stream of patients who eventually will reenter the health care system at some point placing strain when and where it is least needed. But make no mistake about it. While hospitals, health systems, and individual solo and small-group practices are suffering economically, it does not appear that the private health insurance market is mirroring these effects. Many are waiving the costs, co-pays, and deductibles associated with COVID-19, but this pales in comparison to the millions and millions of dollars that these firms are saving by virtue of Americans delaying care while they still collect premiums.[21] The time will come when many will ask why health insurers are not reimbursing policyholders a significant proportion of their 2020 premiums, much like auto insurers have done for drivers who are obviously driving less than in previous years.

We began the COVID-19 pandemic with behavioral nudges designed to keep people at home so that they would not contract or spread COVID-19. The downstream effect of those nudges was to create an environment where both routine and serious health care interventions were sheared to a bare minimum. Getting people back to a "normal" health care equilibrium will be difficult for many reasons as outlined earlier. These reasons combined, together with others that have not been fully elucidated, make those who are staying home fearful of venturing anywhere near a health care facility (and, in some cases, other places, too). We need to find a way, through the use of telehealth, perhaps through the designation of specific hospitals as non-COVID-19 facilities, and urgent health communication strategies to get those who are able to and who are at low risk of contracting COVID-19 to continue with regular and routine care.

Otherwise, it seems in the not-too-distant future, COVID-19 will not be our only problem.

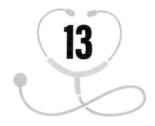

13

Reefer Madness

The choices one makes are limited by the choices one has.

—UNKNOWN

In August 1994, Eric Schlosser wrote an article in *The Atlantic* entitled "Reefer Madness" in which he set out the maddening inconsistencies that govern sentencing guidelines and, ultimately, incarceration in the United States. Astute readers will recognize his name as the same author of *Fast Food Nation: The Dark Side of the All-American Meal* written in 2001. The takeaway from his *Atlantic* article might say more about how armed robbery, rape, and murder are codified in the penal system than anything else, but I digress.

Schlosser, using the state of Indiana as a surrogate marker for the craziness of the American penal system, provides an eye-opening set of statistics for us. He writes that "a person convicted of armed robbery will serve about five years in prison; someone convicted of rape will serve about twelve; and a convicted murderer can expect to spend twenty years behind bars. These figures are actually higher than the figures nationwide: eight years and eight months in prison is the average punishment for an American found guilty of murder."[1] Schlosser then goes on to spotlight the case of Mark Young, a thirty-eight-year-old who acted as a go-between to facilitate the sale of a large amount of marijuana between two parties. He did not actually distribute the marijuana himself nor was there any physical evidence, associated with this arrangement between the two parties that he had brokered, linked to him. Mark Young was sentenced to life in prison without the possibility of parole in 1992.[2]

This chapter is not about marijuana. It is certainly not about marijuana and the American penal system, which, according to Schlosser's 1994 article, suggests that one of every six inmates in the federal prison system—roughly fifteen thousand people—has been incarcerated primarily for a marijuana offense, based on data provided by the Bureau of Prisons and the United States Sentencing Commission.[3] As of June 2020, there were 160,823 offenders incarcerated in the Bureau of Prisons. Of these offenders, 144,121 were serving a sentence for a federal conviction, most commonly for drug offenses ($N = 68,354$).[4] So, while we're not comparing apples to apples, the takeaway from both sets of statistics in 1994 and 2020 is that drug offenses continue to comprise a significant proportion of the incarcerations at a federal level. This chapter is not about whether your recreational use of marijuana is right or wrong. Frankly, I could care less. It's about medical cannabis (which is what I will call it going forward) and why we struggle to incorporate this medicinal agent into our current treatment algorithms for the management of various diseases and ailments. But the historical context of our view on marijuana is an important backdrop for the rest of this chapter because it reveals important, difficult-to-erase biases and societal views.

Medical cannabis has received a mountain of press coverage in recent years for a variety of reasons, ranging from whether it should be legalized to how it should be used (dried, vaporized, or as an oil, etc.) to whether it should be allowed to be advertised or promoted to the general public. All fair questions. The most important question, though, is, Does it work? Isn't this the same question that we ask about every pill or injectable made available to treat a medical condition?

Why does the bar seem to be so much higher for medical cannabis? Look, I can regurgitate the meta-analyses, observational studies, studies with "n's of 10 or 20," and systematic reviews of other authors, but you can easily find them and see the data for yourselves. Here is the cold, hard truth: sometimes medical cannabis works, and sometimes it does not. I've also got some news for you: sometimes your antidepressant works, and sometimes it doesn't. Sometimes your statin works, and sometimes it doesn't. And sometimes your proton pump inhibitor works, and sometimes it doesn't. Given patient heterogeneity and the complex comorbidities that one can present with, it is not surprising that many medical treatments sometimes work and sometimes do not. A principal argument against using medical cannabis has been a variation on the fact that it is not a well-known compound or agent and that we do not have enough experience with it. Bollocks.

The first records of using medical cannabis were in China and India more than two thousand years ago. Dr. Antonio Waldo Zuardi, a leading voice on cannabis research, states in his 2006 article about the history of cannabis use as a medicine, "the use of cannabis as a medicine by ancient Chinese was reported in the world's oldest pharmacopoeia, the *pen-ts'ao ching* which was compiled in the first century of this Era, but based on oral traditions passed down from the time of Emperor Shen-Nung, who lived during the years 2.700 B.C. Indications for the use of cannabis included: rheumatic pain, intestinal constipation, disorders of the female reproductive system, malaria, and others."[5] At about the same time, there are numerous reports of cannabis use in India, where Zuardi also details that the medicinal use of the plant probably began around 1000 BC, when it was routinely used as an analgesic, anticonvulsant, antibiotic, and antispasmodic because it was thought to help in the treatment of numerous conditions. From there, the use of cannabis spread and gained popularity. History shows that medical cannabis was also used in Persia, parts of Arabia in the year AD 1000, in Africa in the fifteenth century, and then on to South America in the sixteenth century. Finally, it made its way into the medicine chest of Western clinicians in the nineteenth and twentieth centuries.[6]

In point of fact, this unknown agent has been in popular medical use for well over two thousand years. But the naysayers point out that, while it has been in use, it has not really been studied in the way we study other therapeutic agents. By that, they mean that there is a paucity of randomized, controlled clinical trials, widely considered the gold standard for judging the efficacy and safety of a novel therapeutic agent for use in humans.

Please. Do not even get me started. First, as of 2018, there were 119 clinical trials assessing the therapeutic potential of cannabinoids registered in the United States alone (figure 18). Call these companies crazy if you want, but the various National Institutes of Health seem to have a similar idea as evidenced by the piles of cash they are throwing at medical cannabis research, too (figure 19). Importantly, let us not forget that the Controlled Substances Act of 1970 classified cannabis as a Schedule I substance, the highest level of drug restriction. The act defines Schedule I substances as those that (1) have a high potential for abuse, (2) have no currently accepted medical use in treatment in the United States, and (3) have a lack of accepted safety for their use under medical supervision. Other substances classified in Schedule I include heroin, LSD, hallucinogenic amphetamine derivatives, and fentanyl derivatives (synthetic opioid analgesics). In juxtaposition to this, Schedule II substances—though they also have a

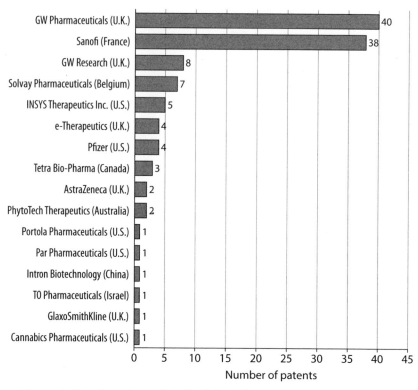

Figure 18. Number of cannabinoid clinical trials registered in the US as of June 2018, by company.

high potential for abuse and may lead to severe psychological or physical dependence—are defined as having a currently accepted medical use and can be prescribed with a controlled substance prescription.[7] In light of this, the ability to effectively conduct research has been hampered—an understatement if ever there was one—by the excruciatingly difficult regulatory barriers for the better part of half a century.

Then there is another practical aspect to conducting randomized trials with cannabis: How exactly do you ensure that trial participants are all getting the same active ingredient? I do not have to remind anyone that cannabis is a plant, and it contains over one

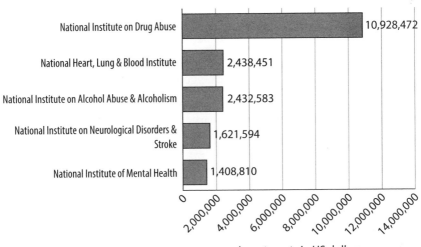

Figure 19. Leading investors in therapeutic cannabis research among the US National Institutes of Health in fiscal year 2015.

hundred different phytocannabinoids (some of which you may recognize: THC and CBD), which are influenced by both plant genetics and growing conditions such that the same strain of cannabis plant can express a different phytocannabinoid profile depending on the location, temperature, light, soil, and stage of its life cycle.[8] I know what you are thinking. If there are 119 clinical trials examining the effects of cannabinoids, isn't that a problem? Possibly. Each study would have its own design and methodology that might have some method of controlling for this variation in theory. My point is not that research is not important or that we do not need to study the drug and its benefits. My point is that we do not need to rely on randomized trials to learn a lot about this agent.

Let's face it, we all appreciate and place tremendous value on the role that randomized trials play in today's world, but here is another reason that they present a real challenge to the optimal use of medical cannabis: given the suffocating inclusion and exclusion criteria required to execute these pivotal studies, the reality is that patients in medical cannabis cohorts would not even mimic what we see in doctors' offices anyway. Who really has a waiting room full of white males, aged from twenty-four to forty-nine, with a normal body mass index, no diabetes, no cardiovascular disease, no smoking history, and a clean mental health history? Actually, this is a problem for all clinical trials—this notion of generalizability. Do the patients in the trial setting reflect the patients that would be receiving this drug in a real-world setting?

The debate about using medical cannabis without the safety net of a randomized, controlled trial to fall back on has, I hope, been largely dismissed as being a must-have. It is definitely a nice-to-have. In case you are still unconvinced, here is an addendum to this whole debate about "traditional" therapeutic agents and medical cannabis: there are lots and lots of drugs that are used off-label. Throughout modern medical history, countless examples of therapeutic agents have been used to treat conditions for which they have not been studied. Skeptical? In 2006, Radley and colleagues used the Intercontinental Medical Statistics (now known as IQVIA) Health National Disease and Therapeutic Index to define prescribing patterns by diagnosis for 160 commonly prescribed drugs. Each reported drug-diagnosis combination was identified as Food and Drug Administration–approved, off-label with strong scientific support, or off-label with limited or no scientific support. To save us all some time, I will cut to the chase. Radley et al. concluded that "off-label medication use is common in outpatient care, and most occurs without scientific support."[9] They go on to say that "we found that about 21% of all estimated uses for commonly prescribed medications were off-label, and that 15% of all estimated uses lacked scientific evidence of therapeutic efficacy."[10] So, this is common practice. It is a weak argument to cite the lack of clinical evidence for medical cannabis as a suitable treatment option for certain patients given the massive amount of off-label use of hundreds of medicines. The very nature of off-label use suggests, to an experienced clinician, that there is a *lack of evidence*, and the care with which clinicians use drugs off-label knowing that the drug has not been studied extensively acts as a natural restrictor on its use. Nobody is suggesting that we figure out a way to put medical cannabis into our drinking water or that we stand on the street corner handing out baggies of cannabis. Ultimately, however, whether it is abortion, assisted suicide, or medical cannabis use, the temperature of the discussion as a social and ethical issue is invariably turned up and the health care conversation tends to get turned down or drowned out.

It is the real-world outcomes and clinical results that count, no? And in the real world, medical cannabis sometimes works. Just like any other medicine. This is not to suggest that future trials that look at the use of medical cannabis in specific patient subpopulations are not important—simply that randomized, controlled trials should not guide our entire thought process on the safety and efficacy of this specific agent. By the way, I am doing a disservice to the well-designed, robust clinical trials that offer sound statistical clues about the potential benefits of medical cannabis in treating certain diseases. It is not as though the entire universe is free of any good studies using medical cannabis. That is simply not true. There is some important work out there. It will take a few more years for us to get the results. But good work is being done. I will be the first to say that medical cannabis is not without its concerns. The deleterious side effects of prolonged medical cannabis use cannot be ignored (respiratory problems, dependency, etc.), and, we should continue to challenge the scientific community and manufacturers to push for research that helps us better understand these factors. No one is advocating for a helter-skelter and scientifically baseless approach to the use of medical cannabis.

Look, there are a lot of issues to discuss when it comes to medical cannabis. But one that has received a good deal of attention and that we ought to pay more attention to is the potential reduction in opioid overdoses with the introduction of medical cannabis as a treatment option for chronic pain. One study has shown that in states where medical cannabis laws exist or have been introduced, there is a 24.8 percent lower mean annual opioid overdose mortality rate compared with states without medical cannabis laws.[11] Another study has demonstrated that, in states where medical cannabis laws exist or have been enacted, the reduction in prescribing opioids is lower by millions of daily doses as compared with states in which there are no medical cannabis laws.[12] The evidence is clear. Medical cannabis can be substituted as a viable treatment approach for chronic pain in patients who might otherwise have been prescribed opioids. Think of the avoidable morbidity and mortality and the costs—both current and downstream—that can be saved. In 2018 alone, almost fifty thousand people died from prescription and synthetic opioid overdoses.[13] Will medical cannabis prevent all of those deaths? Of course not. But even one prevented death is a step in the right direction given all that we know about medical cannabis's safety profile and relatively low addiction or dependency risk.

People tend to get their knickers in a knot because they think that medical cannabis is going to be used for *everything*. What we know is that there is reasonably strong evidence that medical cannabis works in the management of chronic pain, chemotherapy-induced nausea and vomiting, and epilepsy. There is some literature that suggests a possible role in treating anxiety, insomnia, post-traumatic stress disorder, and depression. Everything else is largely unknown, with research, case reports, and real-world utilization still needed to provide further guidance to inform practice management guidelines. Even if we use it in, say, chronic pain management, no one is suggesting that it be used as a first-line treatment option or that it be used in everyone suffering from chronic pain. Most clinicians (and patients) agree that medical cannabis is not going to work for everyone and that it should be used in an appropriate place in the treatment algorithm after other therapies have been tried and failed. If I were a patient who was constantly in pain because of a motor vehicle accident and I had tried other chronic pain medications with no luck, I would want this option made available to me. If I were a clinician who was sick and tired of seeing my patients with diminished quality of life and suffering from constant pain after trying myriad other medications, I would want to offer them this therapy as a last or late resort. Why doesn't everyone see it this way? Do we really want patients suffering from chronic pain, having exhausted every option available to them but one? Is this good care?

Our personal positions on the use of medical cannabis are what they are, but we should understand the growing body of scientific evidence that demonstrates real potential for medical cannabis to help some patients some of the time. My focus on the medical application of cannabis is to dispel the myths around its being an unknown agent with which we have no experience. To dismiss this notion that if there are not robust clinical trials with thousands of patients and tens of thousands of years of patient follow-up, then we simply cannot consider it. To fixate on those patients who are poorly controlled on other treatments and for whom this represents an opportunity to provide symptom relief and perhaps give people some small mark of improved quality of life that they can hang on to for hope. If, after I present these arguments, you still think that medical cannabis has absolutely no place in our treatment paradigm, then that is your prerogative.

We can debate the policy implications of using medical cannabis another day. There are many. Based on the glacial pace of acceptance of medical cannabis in mainstream medicine, it appears we have time. We can decide whether the role of randomized, controlled trials as the underpinning of drug approvals is becoming overemphasized. Or, conversely, whether we ought to make exceptions and find ways to include more real-world outcomes data in our regulatory and drug approval frameworks and stop relying on randomized, controlled trials alone in every scenario.

Ultimately, however, the lens through which I want you to think about the use of medical cannabis is this: Is it a safe and efficacious treatment option in certain patients? Can we help patients who might get back to some level of better health? These are the *only* questions that matter from a health care perspective. And they matter because, perhaps more than "traditional" patients, medical cannabis patients are not obvious. They are not who we think they are, nor do they always turn up where we think they are going to turn up.

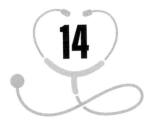

Customer Appreciation

Life can only be understood backwards; but it must be lived forwards.
—Søren Kierkegaard

At a broad level, we really do not know who our patients are, what they look like, and where to find them. We try and tell ourselves otherwise. We insist that we have a handle on these patient factors.

But when we say that we do not know who they are and what they look like, we mean to emphasize that patients may be similar. But they are not the same. Actually, the concept of patients being similar but not the same is an important underpinning that flows into a larger view that we cannot simply compare patients on a basic level. Two patients with cardiovascular disease will possess many similarities, but they are subtly different beyond the obvious characteristics of gender, ethnicity, height, and weight. There is both some observable and unobservable variation between patients. In other words, they possess *heterogeneity*. This is not a term we use outside of health care very often. It is defined

as "that which consists of dissimilar or diverse ingredients or con-
stituents."[1] Most of us are more familiar with its antonym, *homogeneous*. When I was a kid my parents would send me to the store
to buy homogenized milk (before we all knew better and started
buying low-fat or skim milk). I learned early what homogeneous
meant—at least in a food context. But heterogeneous never really
came up in conventional conversation. It does now, sometimes.
We use the word *heterogeneous* in health care. But the clinical use
of the term to describe the approach to disease management is
one thing. The published use of the term to describe the challenges in the interpretation of trial results is another. Even the
recognition of the term in health policy circles is reassuring. But
do we really "get it"?

Do we fundamentally understand that almost everything in
health care is heterogeneous? Do we really get that no two patients
are the same and that they each bring variation to a clinical situation? Maybe that is the easiest part to understand because it is intuitive. It is not a giant leap to understand that, of course, no two
patients are the same because we all have different DNA. But the
rest may not be obvious. That no two doctors are the same and
they, too, vary. And that two different doctors, with the same training and the same years of experience, might read a biopsy result
very differently, which will have tremendous implications for disease management. Do we get that diseases are not the same?
Even those diseases that we think are the same are heterogeneous.
Cancer, as an example, is not a single disease. Cancer is, in fact,
a bunch of different illnesses—each one with its own unique form
of presentation, genetic mutation, progression, manifestation,
and conclusion. Of course, do we get that the drugs we use to treat
these diseases are asymmetrical? Just because two drugs act on the
IL-17 pathway does not mean that the drugs are interchangeable.
And that the side effects of these drugs we use to treat these illnesses are also variable. Some drugs cause gastrointestinal dis-

tress and others cause headaches. Others cause fibromyalgia and some cause dizziness. The efficacy of these therapies for these different patients is not the same. Drugs have different onsets of action and duration of response. Some patients start to see clinical response within days, and others within weeks or months. Some patients will discontinue therapy and relapse while others do not. Do we get that the role of regulatory agencies in drug and device approvals is not the same across many jurisdictions? That the implementation of health policies around the world is not the same. And that the way we pay doctors is not the same. Some are paid a straight salary. Others are paid a fee for service and still others are paid based on a capitated model. And that patent laws around drug molecules are not the same around the world. Hatch-Waxman, march-in rights (the Bayh-Doyle Act), compulsory licensure, and TRIPS are all variations on this theme. Do we get that opinion on how we ought to pay for health care is not the same. And, maybe more germanely, that opinion on who ought to pay for health care is not the same.

Why go through this exhaustive list? Because I really want to drive home a point. Nothing about health care is really, truly directly comparable. And yet we act like it is. Or at least that is what it seems like. We act as though there is a hand-in-glove solution to everything that ails the modern-day health system. Do not let all this talk about precision medicine fool you. That is the exception. The rule is cookie-cutter solutions more often than not. Every company is chasing the same holy grail at the core of their drug development pipeline. Every insurance company offers indistinguishable variations between their insurance plans. Every marketing campaign focuses on the same pillars. Every doctor and allied health care practitioner talks about the same shortcomings of the system they work in (overworked, underpaid, overregulated, and underresourced). Every policy wonk talks about the same levers that need to be pulled (access, cost, equity). Every politician and presidential candidate promises untold riches and funding directed to health care as part of their preelection promise (only to realize that the accounting for what they promised is impossible). And the band marches on. We are literally stuck talking about (with rare exception) the same things we did twenty, thirty, and forty years ago when it came to health care. One big giant echo chamber. How are we going to pay for all of this? Are we training enough doctors or training them the right way? Are insurance companies finding new ways to shift costs to the employers or to patients? How do we maintain a level of innovation that encourages drug companies to discover new drugs? Are patent laws too strict? How do we motivate patients to increase their compliance? How do we address health inequities?

The degree of focus on some of these issues has changed over the last generation. Some have waxed in importance. Some have waned. But they are all still very much present. And there are new problems, too. Do not let management buzzwords like *disruption* fool you. New drugs have been launched and new health policies implemented but they have not been disruptions. They are, what I call, *localized eruptions*. They are felt but not widely. Disruptions impact the health care problem they strive to solve from start to finish. That is to say in an end-to-end manner. Launching a new hepatitis C medication that effectively cures a disease only to have it priced out of reach of most patients or to have insurance companies or pharmacy benefits managers restrict its listing and usage is not a disruption.

To review the lesson: nothing in health care is really without some level of subtle variance, even though we think and act as though it might be. Nothing in health care problem-wise has really changed, even though we think and act as though it has. Then when we have a solution, we tout it as disruptive, even though it is nothing more than a localized eruption that is narrow in focus and effect. Sounds depressing doesn't it? Actually, it's not. It is quite liberating, frankly. Because the answer is right in front of us. Affordability of patented medicines is a problem, you say. OK, why not have different drug prices based on household income? Patent law is a total circus that allows companies to prevent legitimate generic competitors from launching, which in turn drives cost. How about different patent laws for different classes of drugs? Here's an analogy: nobody looks for identical snowflakes or fingerprints. We simply accept that there are none. Maybe we ought to accept that the solution to our health care problems is that there is no single solution to our health care problems. And then we can get on with it.

What about who these patients are? Take a look at figure 20. A lot of people do not know that we spend 27 percent of our total health care dollars on 1 percent of the population. More than half of all spending is on 5 percent of the total population.[2] Who are these people? You might think of them as frequent flyers to borrow a descriptor from another industry. These are the people who have cardiovascular disease and diabetes and respiratory ailments and any other number of chronic ailments. They visit their doctor or the hospital often and use a disproportionately high amount of health care resources—not always receiving the benefit needed or the outcomes desired. Many studies have attempted to examine and explain the nature of health care expenditure, and the results are consistent. Health care expenditure is, of course, driven by technology as newer medicines and medical devices cost more even as we try to introduce wider adoption of generic and biosimilar medicines. Expenditure is certainly linked to supply-side factors, such as ordering more tests and the increasing length of hospital stays.[3] Berk and Monheit point out something interesting and worth taking note of: "While most of our discussion focuses at the high-expenditure tail of the distribution, it is worth noting the extreme stability over time in the amount of resources used by the bottom half of the population." And they go on to

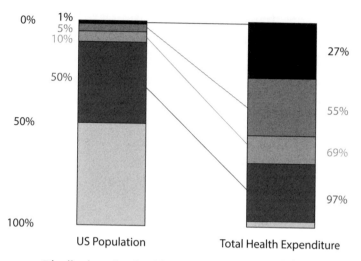

Figure 20. Distribution of US health spending. Adapted from Monheit et al. 2003.

point out that their surveys "all show that the lower 50 percent of the population collectively used about 3 percent of total health care resources. Ideally, one should expect a somewhat skewed distribution; it is certainly not efficient policy for healthy people to be using equivalent services as those who are seriously ill. However, the degree of concentration raises interesting issues: It is clear that the majority of Americans collectively are responsible for only a very small proportion of what is spent (or paid for) on health care."[4] They looked at US health spending over multiple time periods and found that the bottom half of the population consistently accounts for about only 3 percent of total health expenditure.

The issue of how much the top 1 percent, 5 percent, or 10 percent spend is a delicate one. These are sick people. They are vulnerable. Some are elderly and most in need of care. But what else do we know? Well, Dieleman et al. published a wonderful review of US spending on health care just a few years ago. They collected and combined data from government budgets, insurance claims, facility surveys, household surveys, and official US records from 1996 through 2013. Their research team used 183 sources of data to estimate spending for 155 conditions (including cancer, which was disaggregated into 29 conditions). For each record, spending was extracted, along with the age and sex of the patient, and the type of care. Spending was adjusted to reflect the health condition treated, rather than the primary diagnosis.[5] In general, the authors found that there was a tangible increase in health spending between 1996 and 2013—which comes as no surprise to anyone— and that the highest amount of spending was concentrated in areas such as diabetes, heart disease, and chronic pain (lower back and neck).[6] Here is something else that may be surprising: the idea that the frail and elderly (over sixty-five years old) account for most of these expenditures is not entirely accurate. The overall percentage of spending by age on the top fourteen disease conditions shows that those over the age of sixty-five account for 38 percent of spending and those under the age of twenty account for 11 percent of spending across the same fourteen disease conditions (table 7).

Which means that more than half of all spending for these diseases is assigned to people who, by and large, are in the workforce (twenty-one to sixty-four years old). What role does workplace stress play in exacerbating these conditions? What is driving the spending on this "healthiest" segment of our population? If there is a meaningful shift away from helping the twenty-one- to sixty-four-year-old segment with their health care costs, what will the resulting impact be on tax revenue for the government? If employer-based insurance plans continue to shift costs in the form of deductibles and co-pays to the worker and workers continue to struggle to make those minimum payments, will they forego care? Will they reduce their adherence to prescription medications? We know the answers to these questions, and they are not encouraging.

But perhaps these, and other, data remind us that it is not the elderly and frail who are solely responsible for the high health care

Table 7. Personal health care spending by condition

Rank[a]	Aggregated Condition Category	2013[b] Spending (Billions of Dollars), $	Annualized Rate of Change, 1996–2013, %	2013 Spending by Type Care (%)					2013 Spending by Age (%)	
				Ambulatory Care	Inpatient Care	Pharmaceuticals	Emergency Care	Nursing Facility Care	<20 Years	≥65 Years
1	Cardiovascular diseases	231.1	1.2	18.4	57.3	6.2	2.7	15.3	0.9	65.2
2	Diabetes, urogenital, blood, and endocrine diseases	224.5	5.1	31.5	23.0	31.0	4.2	10.3	3.5	42.6
3	Other noncommunicable diseases	191.7	3.1	43.0	11.3	6.5	2.8	3.2	15.3	32.9
4	Mental and substance abuse disorders	187.8	3.7	52.1	19.0	20.9	1.6	6.5	19.8	12.8
5	Musculoskeletal disorders	183.5	5.4	47.7	37.0	6.2	3.3	5.9	1.9	40.0
6	Injuries	168.0	3.3	34.5	33.7	0.7	25.1	6.1	14.1	27.5
7	Communicable, maternal, neonatal, and nutritional disorders	164.9	3.7	21.7	58.1	2.1	6.2	11.8	23.8	36.6
8	Well care	155.5	2.9	28.7	36.5	3.0	0.5	0.1	37.7	5.1
9	Treatment of risk factors	140.8	6.6	35.6	3.5	53.6	1.1	6.2	0.6	50.0

10	Chronic respiratory diseases	132.1	3.7	31.1	26.7	28.4	4.7	9.0	14.5	39.0
11	Neoplasms	115.4	2.5	42.0	51.2	1.0	1.2	4.6	3.0	46.3
12	Neurological disorders	101.3	4.0	26.3	15.0	12.3	3.5	43.0	2.4	58.8
13	Digestive diseases	99.4	2.9	20.6	60.8	5.5	6.4	6.7	6.0	39.3
14	Cirrhosis	4.2	5.1	7.8	88.5	0.0	0.0	3.6	1.3	19.6
	All conditions	2,100.1	3.5	33.6	33.2	13.7	4.9	9.3	11.1	37.9

Source: Adapted from Dieleman et al. (2013).
[a] Ranked from highest spending to lowest spending.
[b] Reported in 2015 US dollars. Uncertainty intervals are reported in the supplement.

costs in America. And that it is not entirely end-of-life care that consumes the most of our health care dollars or that the big, expensive million-dollar heart surgeries are disproportionately skewing the numbers. These data remind us that the young and middle-aged require a significant chunk of the finite health care dollars, too. Dieleman et al. actually broke down these fourteen disease categories into further disaggregated and specific diseases. While some of this disaggregated data that showed a larger percentage of expenditures by younger age category is unsurprising, some of it is also eye-opening. The fact that the percentage of spending on illnesses related to maternal and neonatal diseases is higher in people under twenty years old is expected. But, then, according to the data, we spend at least as much or more on hemoglobinopathies and hemolytic anemias in the young than in the old. The same is true of migraines, appendicitis, other chronic respiratory diseases, and anxiety disorders. Who knew?

When we look at spending by gender in 2013 (figure 21), we see that "estimated spending per person was greater among females than males for age 15 through 64 years and for age 75 years and older, whereas spending per person was greater among males than females for age 65 through 74 years and for younger than 15 years."[7]

I have discussed what are our patients look like and who they are. To be clear, they are as heterogeneous in nature as the rest of health care itself. These patients are not always old and frail but young and hiding in plain sight. But what about the where? Where do we find these patients?

At the annual Harvard Health Care Conference some years ago, I had the pleasure of listening to David Kirchhoff, the CEO of Weight Watchers at the time, speak about the obsession in America around weight loss and the obesity epidemic. Although the years have somewhat impeded my exact memory of the presentation, I distinctly remember starting to think about the people

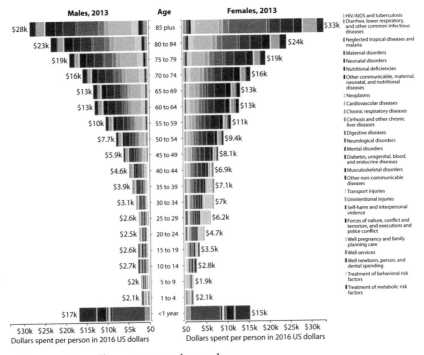

Figure 21. Spending per person, by gender.

who went to these Weight Watchers clinics. I started, in fact, to think about Weight Watchers as a singular organization. As Kirchhoff continued to speak about the revenue and the research and development objectives and the number of employees, I began to wonder if Weight Watchers was a pharmaceutical company disguised as a lifestyle management outfit or a series of obesity clinics disguised as weight loss clinics. Or something in-between. Or none of the above. And then I began to wonder about the people (do we call them patients or consumers?) who attended these Weight Watchers venues. If, in fact, these are patients with real illnesses, comorbid conditions, and psychosocial issues, then don't we need to completely change our model of how we view them if we're going to ensure the provision of services to this patient population?

If we expect that obese people are going to be sitting in our physicians' waiting rooms with their hands neatly folded on their laps waiting for their names to be called so that we can refer them out for bariatric surgery, gastric bypass surgery, sleeve gastrectomy, or even a less (supposedly) invasive approach like the LAP-BAND system, then maybe we're wrong. Maybe, we'll keep on waiting, and the reality is that these patients will not show up in physicians' offices anymore. Maybe we need to ensure that the delivery of care to these patients considers where they actually are and not where we expect them to be.

What about mental health patients? Another classic example of assuming where the patients will be instead of actually knowing where they are. If I asked you to name the largest mental health institution in North America (a.k.a. the largest mental hospital), what would you guess? McLean Hospital? Johns Hopkins? Maybe New York Presbyterian? You'd be wrong on all three counts. The largest mental hospital in North America is Cook County Jail.[8]

A jail.

If we're going to change the slope of the mental health curve and bring meaningful interventions to this group of patients, then we ought to know where a significant majority of them are—no? If your argument is something along the lines of *are we really going to change the way we deliver mental health services based on a cohort of people who are behind bars?*, then you know better than that. You know that the incarcerated population is simply a surrogate marker for any disenfranchised population segment that has unequal access to mental health services.

There are, of course, plenty of other examples of disease states where patients are not lined up neatly waiting for the provision of services—disease states where the lines are blurred between where we think patients are and where they actually are. And the point of these examples is that we need to inject, within our health policy thinking, significant brainpower aimed at better understanding where patients are and, more important, how to deliver the services they need where they are. Instead of continuously trying to devise ways of driving patients to the provider, the goal should be to work toward a model of geolocation of care. We have become adept at throwing around buzzwords such as *point of care* and *point of diagnosis* without stopping to think that this point is not a fixed point (as the fixed-point theorems of mathematics might suggest). This point is not a point at all. It is a series of points. And all of these individual points making up this larger point of care represent patients.

We've spent so much time debating and discussing the cost of therapies and how we need to ensure price transparency to control costs and how we need to hold pharmaceutical companies accountable and get a peek into that black box of pricing. We've gutted ourselves with the angst of trying to prevent cost shifting from happening in the private payer market with higher co-pays, deductibles, annual caps, and lifetime caps. Everywhere you turn, someone wants to talk about cost and every think tank has a slant on the topic. Here's a sobering thought: Can you imagine how much we'd be spending on health care if we actually knew where all the patients were?

Make no mistake. In the end, knowing where all these patients are and what they look like is about more than cost and access. It's also about understanding who these patients influence and who influences them.

15

Under the Influence

I may not have gone where I intended to go, but I think I have ended up where I needed to be.

DOUGLAS ADAMS, *The Long Dark Tea-Time of the Soul*

Traditional and social media are changing health care. And probably not in the way you're thinking.

It is not entirely uncommon for consumer-packaged goods companies or luxury retailers to pay Facebook, YouTube, or Instagram "stars" to endorse and use their brands. Typically, these individuals have the profile of a customer that the manufacturer or retailer wishes to target, with one mandatory characteristic and requirement: they also have tens of thousands (if not more) of followers on social media. These people are commonly known as *influencers*.

In health care, the trend of using patient influencers has started to gain significant traction over the past few years. These patient influencers are becoming more ubiquitous. Much of the mainstream perspective on the role of patient influencers focuses on whether there are inherent conflicts of interest in using existing patients to speak to other patients or prospective patients, whether this activity transgresses the tight rules around direct-to-consumer advertising and, pragmatically, how we can control the influencer's user generated content. But rarely do we discuss the policy, public health, and behavioral implications of this growing trend.

As Diaz-Martin and colleagues write in a recent article published in *Frontiers in Psychology*,

> in the past health information was created by doctors and used by patients, nowadays these lines become blurry as patients are increasingly in charge of their own health, collaborate with healthcare professionals rather than passively receive information from them and even create their own health recommendations for other users. This shift toward more informed, empowered and enabled patients is both desired and handy and has clear implications on the ways people interact with healthcare professionals and the healthcare system itself.[1]

The shift toward more informed, empowered, and enabled patients is certainly desirable, but, as I proffered earlier in chapter 6, "The Rating Game," on the role of platforms such as Yelp and Care Dash that empowerment can have unintended consequences.

Sun et al. describe these influencers as "health e-mavens" and make clear that these individuals are characterized by two distinct, primary online behaviors: health information acquisition and transmission. In other words, these influencers or mavens are unique for both information seeking and sharing behaviors where health information *acquisition* consists of two specific activities, health information tracking and consulting, and health information *transmission* comprises information sharing and online posting activities.[2] Their analysis also revealed that individuals who were female or had a higher education level were more likely to be health e-mavens and that both health status and health insurance were positive predictors of health e-mavenism, suggesting that individuals with more health problems and more health insurance plans were more likely to become active users of online information.[3]

In truth, no matter the definition, we have known about influencers for years. Malcolm Gladwell described them in his landmark book, *The Tipping Point: How Little Things Can Make a Big Difference* published in 2000. Gladwell introduced us to "connectors" and "mavens." Connectors are, well, in the habit of connecting people as one would surmise. However, it is not only the simple act of connecting that is important but, as Gladwell states, the sheer number of connections that these individuals can bring together. Mavens, in contrast, are not about people and connections. Mavens share knowledge and spread information.[4] In essence, patient influencers are part connector and part maven, which is what makes them incredibly valuable to pharmaceutical companies who are now paying such influencers to share their experiences about products and raise awareness about disease states.

I submit to you that being an uber-connector and an uber-maven is not enough. One other factor makes these influencers incredibly persuasive and valuable beyond the fact that they know a lot of people and are good at sharing information: they look like us. Not necessarily from a physical point of view—although that helps but from an emotional, psychosocial, and experiential point of view. The academic literature has reinforced what we already knew intuitively, which is that we feel more closely aligned to people who are similar to us and that we are predisposed to, more likely than not, find such people credible. Herein lies the value of the influencer. It is not important at all that the influencer be famous. I would argue it matters more that they are not. It may not even be important that an influencer is acting in an official capacity on behalf of a brand. Informal influencing is rampant. Passing around nutrition and exercise advice at your neighbor's barbecue is commonplace. Today, that exchange of advice in an informal setting has multiplied to the extent that it is routine to hear friends and family members talking about what helps their lower back pain and how they deal with side effects of common medications. You may not consider this patient influencing, but it is. It most definitely is. And social media has weaponized this.

Here is a silly but relatable example. In the late 1990s when the two biggest athletes on the planet were Michael Jordan and Tiger Woods, we saw them hawking goods on television like Hanes underwear and Buick cars. Predictably, the impact of their respective endorsements on driving consumer demand was, well, infinitesimal.[5] Not because the brands were crappy. Or that they were bad influencers. But because they did not "look" like most of the Hanes and Buick target audiences. What was more of a disconnect for consumers was the experiential aspect of the endorsement. Nobody actually believed that a twenty-two-year-old man who had just won the Masters golf tournament and could drive any car in the world would walk into a Buick dealership and pick out a Buick Regal for himself. Nobody believed that Michael Jordan, who was legendary for his $5,000 custom-made suits, was going to slip on a pair of $4 Hanes underwear purchased from the local Kmart down the street.

It is this hallmark of having "walked a mile in your shoes" that draws us to all influencers, including those of the patient persuasion. They know what we are feeling, what we have gone through, and what to expect. When they describe the pain and the limitations of simple daily activities associated with the illness that we, too, have experienced, it is as if they live inside of us. When they describe the debilitating side effects of therapy, it is as if they speak for us. And when they advocate for better access and lower prices for patients with the same condition that we have, it is as if they know us. They are connectors and mavens. But they are also part prophet and part therapist.

The advent of influencing as an entity unto itself certainly did not start with social media, and it is not restricted to familiar platforms such as Facebook, Instagram, and TikTok. It started, and continues today, with television and public awareness messages such as "Ask your doctor" campaigns. But it has also mutated to include full-blown endorsements of prescription medications from instantly recognizable faces. In 1958, Milton Berle became one of the first celebrities to promote a pharmaceutical drug, according to a review published in the *American Journal of Public Health*, when the comedian joked about his use of a depressant called Miltown, from the drug manufacturer Carter Products. And from there it continued throughout the 1960s, '70s, and '80s, as pharmaceutical companies paid popular writers such as Lawrence Galton and Donald Cooley to write hundreds of articles promoting drugs, according to the *AJPH* review.[6]

And then two landmark policy changes occurred.

According to Drugwatch, a consumer advocacy group based in Orlando, Florida, that works to educate the public on dangerous drugs and medical devices and to empower consumers to assert their legal rights, "in 1985, the FDA lifted a ban on direct-to-consumer advertising, establishing standards that stated companies had to communicate a balance of benefits, risks and side effects of drugs in ads and in 1997, the FDA relaxed its rules, allowing pharmaceutical companies to advertise to consumers by mentioning less information about side effects if they told consumers where they could find more information about the drugs." Thus, opened the floodgates of more commercials advertising the potential benefits of prescription drugs, as well as using celebrities to get the message about these potential benefits across to sufferers and patients. This was the precursor to the modern-day use of influencers.

There was, and continues to be, fierce backlash. Opponents argue that these thinly veiled, quasi-altruistic attempts to paint the use of celebrity influencers as simply a means to increase awareness about diseases and conditions that have an incredibly high burden of illness and for which there is little mainstream reporting is nothing more than a sham. If that was true, then why do we not see similar appeals for the same conditions from generic drug manufacturers, says Dr. Michael Carome, the director of Public Citizen's Health Research Group.[7]

Others have pointed out that celebrity influencing can have deleterious effects, albeit unintended and unbeknownst to the influencer. Model Lauren Hutton was hired by Wyeth to advocate for a discussion of hormonal therapies between a woman and her doctor. The long-term evidence later demonstrated that hormone replacement therapy could increase the risk of developing breast cancer, and Pfizer (Wyeth's parent company) settled lawsuits totaling almost $1 billion related to the use of its hormone replacement drug Prempro.[8] In 2000, Bruce Jenner and Dorothy Hamill (former US Olympians) were both hired by Merck to promote the benefits of Vioxx, a COX-2 inhibitor introduced by Merck in 1999 as an effective, safer alternative to non-steroidal anti-inflammatory drugs for the treatment of pain associated with osteoarthritis.[9] Investigative reporting and subsequent litigation by tens of thousands of plaintiffs revealed that scientists and executives at Merck were aware that the drug might adversely affect the cardiovascular system by altering the ratio of prostacyclin to thromboxane, which act in opposition, balancing blood flow and clotting.[10] Nobody is suggesting that Lauren Hutton, Bruce Jenner, or Dorothy Hamill should have been aware of the long-term safety concerns with these molecules. Rather, the point is that endorsement and influence on the use of specific therapies or, at a broader level, can have consequences.

There is the obvious pushback that, independent of long-term adverse events and pseudo-selling-disguised-as-awareness campaigns, there is no fundamental way to control user generated content, whether or not it is celebrity driven. The most famous example of this is with Kim Kardashian and her Diclegis Instagram post. In 2015, Kardashian posted an endorsement of a morning sickness medication without all the usual disclaimers about the safety risks associated with its use. The manufacturer behind the morning sickness medication received a stern warning letter from the US Food and Drug Administration but the damage (depending on your perspective) had been done: four hundred ninety thousand likes and millions of retweets, shares, and free public relations for the medication. In a world that lives in real time, it is almost impossible to prevent this kind of misbehavior. And this says nothing of the posts, tweets, and endorsements generated by non-celebrities— the type of content generated from real patients mind you, but that does not receive the glare and oversight of federal regulators. What happens when Jane Smith from Anywhere, USA, promotes a drug like Kim Kardashian did? You might argue that Jane probably has one-millionth the social media followers of Kardashian, so there is really nothing to worry about. But when you stop and think about it, you realize there are tens of thousands of Jane Smiths, and each one is either formally or informally influencing.

So, the public health and policy learning from this growing trend of using patient influencers is that we may drive unnecessary health care utilization. One of the best public databases in the United States for looking at the online habits of patients, the Health Information and National Trends Survey, shows that people are increasingly using the internet to seek health information and that they are increasingly comfortable with it as their first option for potential answers. For those who are undiagnosed, we may be driving them to their primary care providers needlessly seeking diagnosis through the validation of weakly-related symptoms to some illness. For those who are already diagnosed, we may be driving these patients to seek more expensive treatment options as they see patient influencers with their same illness using treatment modalities that provide higher quality of life and wonder, What about me? These patients now start badgering their doctor about "the thing I saw on TV" or the "thing my friend posted on Facebook."

The question that always keeps us up at night when it comes to technology and health care is whether any redeeming aspect of this situation can be harnessed to solve health care's big problems. There just might be one: the ability for patient influencers to aggregate opinions and experiences of patients and potential patients is tantalizing. We may soon have incredibly rich insights into traditional black box topics as a result of these patient influencers and their networks, topics such as pharmacovigilance using user generated content collected through patient influencers. Imagine the ability to better understand whether the reaction to a biologic medication injection described in (almost) real time is a simple injection site reaction or a more alarming allergic reaction. Or being able to ascertain patient compliance and persistence to therapy. Or comprehending the packaging and design of your pill bottle or blister pack to better meet the needs of elderly people who struggle with the simple daily task of taking their medicines. Imagine, for a host of pediatric diseases, the ability to aggregate feedback on efficacy, safety, quality of life, and other important dimensions using younger influencers who can build strong bonds with patients of their similar age and background. While there are challenges with such social listening platforms, such as the inability to distinguish between ambiguous or ill-defined terminology, the artificial intelligence and deep learning algorithms being developed may soon get us there.

Barring a major regulatory or legal barrier, it seems reasonable to believe that patient influencers—both formal and informal—are here to stay. While sharing disease and product information, connecting patients with one another, and generally providing an avenue for patients to gain important information about disease management are all incredibly important features of this growing trend, perhaps its best application will be revealed through the adoption of new public health and policy guidelines. What these new public health and policy guidelines end up being is anyone's guess, but it will involve the use of real-world evidence—a form of data that can be incredibly useful. But, at the same time, not all data are created equal.

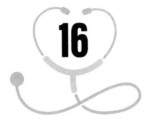

Data Dump

Ever tried. Ever failed. No matter. Try again. Fail again. Fail better.

—SAMUEL BECKETT

Understanding the data we are looking at is critically important in epidemiology. But understanding *how* the data were collected and their limitations might be equally important.

Which data should we trust, and which can we throw out? Is the gold standard of the randomized controlled trial, also known as the RCT, really the gold standard? Do we rely on it way too much to inform policy and clinical decision making? What other forms of data collection are valuable tools?

The most commonly accepted definition of epidemiology comes from McMahon and Pugh: "Epidemiology is the study of the distribution and determinants of disease frequency in man."[1] Pay special attention to the words *distribution* and *determinants* because the distribution of disease is uncovered through what are called descriptive studies, such as cross-sectional studies, case reports, or ecologic studies in which we are really only looking at the *who, what, when,* and *where* of disease. However, the determinants of disease are best elucidated through analytic studies, such as observational (case control or cohort) and intervention studies (RCTs) in which we are searching for the *why* of disease.

Each study type brings with it its own unique approach to data analysis. Ecologic studies use data from entire populations to compare disease frequencies among different groups during the same period of time or among the same population at different times. But the problem with this staple epidemiological study is that people forget that the data are of populations and not individuals, which leads to the ecologic fallacy of incorrectly assuming that an association on a population level reflects an association on an individual level. The other big problem is that we erroneously assign some level of causation in ecologic studies, forgetting of course that association is not causation. Two classic examples of this association versus causation confusion come from ecological studies a half-century apart. In the 1950s, researchers were interested in exploring the risk factors for coronary heart disease in a population-level data set. They found strong relationships with age, per capita smoking rates, diet, alcohol consumption, and other factors. This all makes perfect sense. But the strongest risk factor from this data set was the per capita ownership of color television sets. Come again? And in a non-health example from 2009, researchers commissioned by the real estate sector were interested in exploring the benefits of home ownership with the aim of trying to convince people to buy more homes. They found what they thought was a really strong association, one that would be convincing: children living in owned homes (vs. rented) were less likely to drop out of high school. Since one of the largest segments of homeowners are families with children, this was sure to be a big driver of increasing home ownership. What parent does not want to see their child complete high school? If home ownership could help a child stay in school, then it was obvious that home sales would soon skyrocket. What the researchers did not count on was that there was a variable in their data set that had a stronger association with children not dropping out of school: family car ownership.[2]

Ownership of color TV sets and cars do not, as you realize, have any causal relationship with coronary heart disease or school dropout rates. Neither of these variables cause a person to develop heart disease or stay in school. Rather, they both are surrogate markers for the true causal variable.[3] Maybe people who own TV sets are wealthier and because they are wealthier, they eat richer foods and exercise less. Because they eat richer foods and have a more sedentary lifestyle, perhaps it is income that is the true causal variable that predicts coronary heart disease risk and not TV ownership. The same is also true of the real estate example. Income is the true causal variable. Families that own cars have more disposable income, which allows them to, perhaps, afford tutors and computers and extra resources that help children achieve higher grades. It is not car ownership per se that is causally related to high school dropout rates.

Another type of important descriptive study is the case report or case series. Case reports are defined as "the scientific documentation of a single clinical observation and have a time-honored and rich tradition in medicine and scientific publication. A case report is a powerful tool to disseminate information on unusual clinical syndromes, disease associations, unusual side effects to therapy, or response to treatment."[4] They are the most basic type of descriptive study, but we must, again, be aware of a striking limitation: there is no comparison group in a case report. Case reports (or case series) are excellent tools for raising a hypothesis that can be further elucidated in the environment of an analytic study with an appropriate comparison group.[5]

The last type of descriptive study that informs us on who, what, when, and where of the distribution of disease is the cross-sectional study. Cross-sectional data measure the health outcomes in a population at a single point in time or over a short period of time. The fundamental problem with cross-sectional data are that we are not always clear on the temporal nature of the relationship—a chicken and egg problem. What came first, the exposure or the outcome? If drinking milk is associated with the development of peptic ulcers, is that the case because milk causes the ulcer or because ulcer sufferers drink milk to relieve their symptoms?[6]

Now, let's talk about analytic studies, which are fundamentally designed to improve on the limitations of the descriptive study. Analytic studies produce data that look at individuals (unlike ecological studies, which look at populations). They have a comparator group (unlike case reports or case series, which do not). Analytic studies also have an appropriate time sequence (unlike cross-sectional studies, which can confuse the interpretation of the exposure and the outcome because we do not know what came first or second). Finally, analytic studies all have adequate control of confounding (which is an issue for all studies) and which I will discuss later.

Two types of analytic studies are observational and intervention. Each is different based on the exposure variable, but at the heart of it, in an observational study we have no control over when the study participants have been exposed. Let us say we are interested in the relationship between an exposure—alcohol—and an outcome—liver disease. In an observational study, the alcohol consumption happens without our involvement. We are merely observing the natural order of the world. Based on the criteria for our analysis, participants may be selected into an observational study based on the outcome (liver disease), in which case we would call this a case-control observation study. We would observe people with liver disease and look at their exposure to alcohol (i.e., how much did they drink, how often, and for how long). Participants may have been selected into an observational study based on the exposure variable (alcohol consumption; yes or no) and followed over time to see who developed liver disease. This is known as a cohort study.[7]

The advantages of a case-control study are clear. Because we are selecting people on the basis of the outcome (liver disease), it is easy to identify an adequate number of diseased people. In addition, the cost to execute a study of this type is relatively cheap compared to other types of study design, and with a case-control study, we can evaluate multiple exposures or risk factors at the same time. For cohort studies, the advantages are also worth mentioning: We can correctly line up the exposure and the outcome because we have the right temporal sequence. We generally have really good information on exposure status because participants are observed based on the presence or absence of the exposure to begin with. We can literally observe the number of drinks and the frequency of alcohol consumption without having to rely on patient-reported insights or faulty memory. We can also study several outcomes associated with a single exposure. Let us not forget that cohort studies are expensive and time consuming as we must follow participants until the outcome has occurred. Liver disease can take years and years before it manifests, and this lengthy follow-up can give rise to another major problem with cohort studies, which is the ability to deal with the loss of patients due to this lengthy follow-up.[8] Patients move away or die (unrelated to liver disease) or simply stop coming in for their study visits. How does that affect our ability to interpret the relationship between the exposure and the outcome? So, observational data in the form of case-control and cohort studies are valuable and informative but not without their flaws.

The gold standard of analytic studies is the intervention study, also known as the randomized controlled trial, or RCT. As Vinay

Prasad, a leading voice in the push to recognize both the importance and the limitations of various clinical trial designs, states "well designed, adequately powered randomized controlled trials are rightfully considered the highest form of evidence on which to base treatment and diagnostic decisions, minimizing potential biases, particularly confounding, that plague alternate, lesser forms of evidence."[9]

In an RCT, we have the greatest degree of control over the exposure. We actually allocate the exposure to study participants as opposed to other types of trial designs where we simply observe what the natural world order gives us. We can detect small to moderate-sized effects. Importantly, because we randomize all the participants, we can minimize the potential for bias. But RCTs are not perfect. Not even close. It is not that I am anti-RCT. The RCT is the foundation of data interpretation, but it is not the only tool. It, too, has its warts and bruises. Talarico and colleagues showed that among cancer drugs approved by the US Food and Drug Administration (FDA) between 1995 and 2002, demographics of patients were strikingly different from cancer patients in the United States. While the proportions of patients aged ≥65, ≥70, and ≥75 years were 60 percent, 46 percent, and 31 percent, respectively, among cancer patients in the United States, these age groups comprised only 36 percent, 20 percent, and 9 percent of patients in registration trials ($P < .001$).[10] In an eye-opening indictment of the challenges associated with RCTs, Hilal and colleagues asked a simple question: "How often are anticancer drugs approved by the FDA based on clinical trials with the following limitations: nonrandomized design, lack of demonstrated survival advantage, inappropriate use of crossover, or the use of suboptimal control arms?" The answer was, perhaps, unsurprisingly alarming. The authors reported having evaluated a total of 187 trials, leading to 176 approvals for seventy-five distinct novel anticancer drugs by the FDA. Sixty-four (34%) were single-arm clinical trials, and 123 (66%) were RCTs. A total of 125 (67%) had at least one limitation in the domains of interest; 60 of the 125 trials (48%) were RCTs. Of all 123 randomized clinical trials, 37 (30%) lacked overall survival benefit, 31 (25%) had a suboptimal control, and 17 (14%) used crossover inappropriately. In total, two-thirds of cancer drugs are approved based on clinical trials with limitations in at least one of four essential domains, the authors concluded.[11] There are many who propose that pragmatic clinical trials may be more meaningful than RCTs. While we accept that RCTs provide high-quality evidence about the potential benefits and harms of medical interventions, the insights derived are not always relevant to clinical practice. RCTs are, by virtue of their inclusion and exclusion criteria, a collation of homogeneous patient populations and attempt to answer questions of efficacy under ideal conditions. Pragmatic trials, on the other hand, "compare two or more medical interventions that are directly relevant to clinical care or health care delivery and strive to assess those interventions' effectiveness in real-world practice."[12] Importantly, pragmatic trials focus on whether an intervention works in the setting of usual care, and they address practical aspects of care such as cost and access with the overarching goal of achieving generalizability of results.[13]

In the world of descriptive and analytic studies, there are certain words that force us to pay attention, such as *randomize* and *bias*. There are other words, too: *rerum cognoscere causas*. This phrase translates as "to know the causes of things." It is the basis and impetus of public health. But epidemiologists also have a different word for it: *causal inference*.

Let's unpack some of these important concepts such as randomization, causal inference, and bias.

What exactly is randomization, and what does it do? Broglio writes that "the most compelling way to establish that an intervention definitively causes a clinical outcome is to randomly allocate patients into treatment groups. Randomization helps to ensure that a certain proportion of patients receive each treatment and that the treatment groups being compared are similar in both measured and unmeasured patient characteristics."[14] Basically, we want to eliminate any potential differences between all groups in an RCT such that they are effectively the same or identical. Unfortunately, the RCT is not always easy to execute because of cost, time-to-completion, ethical concerns, and other issues.

What about causal inference? Assume that we have an exposure denoted by A and an outcome denoted by Y. I ask you, Does A cause Y? How can we be sure that A alone caused Y and that some other variable didn't have a hand in this relationship between A and Y? Let's put this in practical heath care terms. Does drinking one to two glasses of wine per day result in a lower risk of heart disease as compared to people who don't drink one to two glasses of wine per day? Is a little bit of wine beneficial? Or are drinkers of one to two glasses of wine more affluent and able to maintain a healthy lifestyle? Using a different scenario, do people who get the flu vaccine have a lower mortality rate than those who don't get vaccinated? Does the vaccine increase survival? Or are those who get vaccinated less sick than those who don't get vaccinated?[15]

Here's another way to look at it. Take a look at the fictitious scenarios in table 8 and think about it for a brief moment. Do you think the pill caused John's death in scenario 1? And what about scenario 2? Most likely you would say that the pill did, indeed, cause John's death in scenario 1 but did not have an effect on Jim's survival in scenario 2. Why is this the case? Because the outcomes are different for John in scenario 1 and the same for Jim in scenario 2. We tend to compare the outcome when an exposure is present versus when it is absent. If the outcomes are different, we say that the exposure has a causative effect. In John's case, the act of taking the pill or not taking the pill resulted in a different outcome.

Table 8. Fictitious scenarios of causal inference

Scenario 1	Scenario 2
On April 1, John took a red pill. Five days later he died.	On April 1, Jim did not take a red pill. Five days later he was alive.
Had John not taken the red pill (all other things being equal), five days later he would have been alive.	Had Jim taken the red pill (all other things being equal), five days later he would have been alive.

Source: Adapted from Hernan lecture.

For Jim, the action of taking the pill or not taking the pill resulted in the same outcome.[16]

While causal inference, which attempts to explain the effect of an exposure or treatment on an outcome, is the backbone of much of what we do in public health, we often get tripped up by confounding.

Confounding is a type of bias that arises when we make causal inferences based on non-comparable groups. We can't have people of different ages, different genders, or different baseline health status in different groups and then attempt to draw some meaningful causative conclusion about those two groups. The two groups are, by definition, different. We can say that there is an association between the exposure and the outcome in these groups. But we cannot say that the exposure causes the outcome, unless we control for those differences.

We are right back at square one. But we still need to make policy decisions. We still need to know whether to treat or not to treat. We have to use observational studies (e.g., case controls or cohort studies) and data to guide and inform our approach to disease management. In using an observational approach, we must know how to tell whether a variable is a confounder.

Let's look at a simple example in the observational world: the case of whether age is a confounder for the relationship between coronary heart disease (the exposure) and death (the outcome).

Table 9. Criteria for assessing confounding

---

1. The covariate of interest must be *independently* associated with the outcome.
2. The covariate of interest must be associated with the exposure.
3. The covariate *cannot* be on the causal pathway between the exposure and the outcome.

For a variable to be considered a confounder, three criteria must be met (table 9).

1. Age must be independently associated with death. And it is. Older people are more likely to die than younger people, irrespective of whether they have heart disease (hence, the importance of the words *independently associated with*).
2. Age must be associated (although not independently) with coronary heart disease. And it is. Older people tend to have a greater prevalence of heart disease than younger people.
3. Age cannot be on the causal pathway between coronary heart disease and death. Having coronary heart disease does not cause one to age, which, in turn, leads one to die.

Our three criteria are met. And, as a result, age is a confounder in our observational study of the effect of coronary heart disease on the risk of death.

Why am I bothering to explain all this background on different studies and get into the weeds on descriptive versus analytic? Why bother waxing poetic about causal inference and confounding and bothering to show rudimentary examples of each of these in practice? Because data are everywhere in health care, whether they appear in a scientific journal or a mainstream media article. The more we understand about the types of data, the power of observational data, the incredibly important role of randomization, and data collection limitations, the more likely we are to continue to advance the cause of obtaining a better understanding in how to make them more meaningful and because we are reminded that data, as a tool, work when we are careful and measured in our approach. And they do not, when we are sloppy. As obvious as these platitudes and clichés about the importance of data are, we forget too quickly that the importance of data is not solely an academic exercise related to better understanding confounding and causation versus association. Data, in fact, are a coveted aspect of health care that drives better care management, but the darker side to data coalesces around duplicity and misrepresentation.

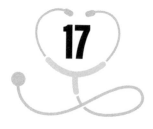

Catch Me If You Can

Rather fail with honor than succeed by fraud.

—SOPHOCLES

We bemoan the rising costs of drugs and devices in the overall health system cost equation. We fret about the cost of labor (i.e., physician salaries). We worry about the increasingly expensive and complex insurance options available to patients.

What we should really be concerned about is the rising cost of health care fraud. By cost, I mean actual cost as well as the human cost of one's health status. Fraud involves everyone: provider fraud, patient fraud, industry fraud. Everyone is implicated. The irony of the situation is that as we develop increasingly complex and sophisticated tools and platforms to drive better care delivery and improve outcomes, our ability to produce equally effective and technologically advanced fraud has kept pace. The Department of Health and Human Services and the Department of Justice's *Health Care Fraud and Abuse Control Program Annual Report for Fiscal Year 2018* shows that the Department of Justice (DOJ) opened 1,139 new criminal health care fraud investigations and that federal prosecutors filed criminal charges in 572 cases involving 872 defendants in which 497 defendants were convicted of health care fraud-related crimes during the year.[1] Just let that sink in for a moment. That is an average of more than three new criminal investigations per day for the whole year. And that is the fraud we know about and the fraud that we have the manpower to chase down. The Federal Bureau of Investigation estimates that fraudulent billings to public and private health care programs make up 3 percent to 10 percent of total health spending;[2] based on current health expenditure data, this would amount to approximately $100 billion at the low end. For those of us who are not accustomed to thinking about the health care system through this lens, let me paint a picture for you. If you took the total cost of care for all the uninsured people in a single year in America and added it up, it would be close to $100 billion or slightly more.[3] In case the math is not obvious, the aggregate total of health care fraud could pay for the medical care of the uninsured in America each and every year. What does this non-corporate fraud look like (tables 10 and 11)?[4]

Table 10. Common examples of provider fraud

- Billing for services not actually performed
- Falsifying a patient's diagnosis to justify tests, surgeries, or other procedures that aren't medically necessary
- Misrepresenting procedures performed to obtain payment for noncovered services, such as cosmetic surgery
- Upcoding—billing for a more costly service than the one actually performed
- Unbundling—billing each stage of a procedure as if it were a separate procedure
- Accepting kickbacks for patient referrals
- Waiving patient co-pays or deductibles and overbilling the insurance carrier or benefit plan
- Billing a patient more than the co-pay amount for services that were prepaid or paid in full by the benefit plan under the terms of a managed care contract

Table 11. Common examples of consumer fraud

- Filing claims for services or medications not received
- Forging or altering bills or receipts
- Using someone else's coverage or insurance card

Non-corporate fraud is pretty run-of-the-mill stuff. But then there is also the sexy stuff. The front-page stuff, for example, data breaches and hacking that demand a ransom or threaten to reveal the health records of millions of consumers. Over forty-one million patient records were breached in 2019, with a single hacking incident affecting close to twenty-one million records as described by Protenus, a health care compliance analytics firm, that looked at data breach incidents disclosed to the Department of Health and Human Services.[5] At the top of the list of these breaches are hacking incidents—particularly ransomware—which are the most common, accounting for 58 percent of the total number of breaches in 2019. These breaches are used for everything from fraudulently billing for or receiving care to filling bogus prescriptions to purchasing items (figure 22). As Protenus reports, "there were incidents of hackers attempting to extort money from patients whose records were exposed, not just the affected healthcare organization. In one incident in Florida, hackers sent ransom demands to a number of the affected patients, threatening the public release of their photos and personal information unless unspecified ransom demands are negotiated and met."[6] Then there are incidents such as the massive security breach at American Medical Collection Agency (AMCA), a third-party billing collections firm in which at least four clinical labs, including Quest Diagnostics and LabCorp, were affected by AMCA's security breach, which exposed the personal data of at least twenty million patients. The breach was discovered when analysts discovered

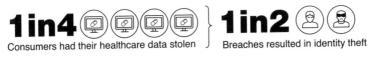

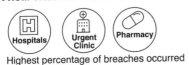

STOLEN DATA USED TO:	37%	35%	26%	26%	12%
	Purchase items	Fraudulently bill for care	Fraudulently receive care	Fraudulently fill prescriptions	Access/modify health records

Figure 22. Health care data breaches among US consumers, 2017. Adapted "One in Four US Consumers Have Had Their Healthcare Data Breached, Accenture Survey Reveals," Accenture.com, https://newsroom.accenture.com/subjects /technology/one-in-four-us-consumers-have-had-their-healthcare-data-breached -accenture-survey-reveals.htm.

patient information, including dates of birth, Social Security numbers, and physical addresses, for sale on the dark web.[7] Scary stuff.

According to a global survey conducted by the Ponemon Institute along with IBM Security, in-depth interviews with nearly five hundred companies across seventeen sectors that experienced a breach revealed that health care data breaches cost, on average, $6.45 million per breach. Health care organizations pay over $400 per lost or stolen record on average, which is nearly three times higher than the non–health care industry average of around $150 per lost or stolen record.[8]

The numbers are staggering, and the scope of the problem is mind-bending. The solution is most certainly not one dimensional. I'm not even sure there is a solution. This might be a case of bending and not breaking. A $100 billion problem (at the low end) does not lend itself to easy fixes and band-aid solutions. The high-profile, front-page fraud is the exception and not the rule. It's the day-to-day provider fraud, such as billing for services not rendered, and patient fraud, such as attempting to recover payment for services not received, that are the bigger problem. And it is a bigger problem because it is harder to ferret out and enforce. There are close to one million active, licensed physicians in the United States and hundreds of millions of patient interactions that potentially could lead to either provider or patient fraud. Perhaps we must accept a certain level of fraud in the system as the cost of doing business.

But what about industry fraud? As in Apple slowing down iPhones or Volkswagen gaming their emissions data or Google skewing search results and banks having manipulated foreign exchange markets. It seems like everyone is cheating these days. And the pharmaceutical industry is no exception.

In an analysis that chronicles twenty-five years' worth of pharmaceutical industry settlements and court judgments, Public Citizen found that, from 1991 through 2015, 373 settlements were reached between the federal and state governments and pharmaceutical manufacturers, totaling $35.7 billion.[9] And this is just in the United States. If we include worldwide financial penalties that have been levied against pharmaceutical companies, the aggregate number is staggering. Perhaps you are not convinced that this happens in other jurisdictions. Well, Pfizer was fined a record £84.2 million by the UK's competition regulator after the price charged to the National Health Service for an anti-epilepsy drug was increased by up to 2,600 percent. The Competition and Markets Authority, issuing this fine, said the "extraordinary price rises have cost the NHS and the taxpayer tens of millions of pounds."[10] And in 2018 an arrangement between Roche and Novartis to channel demand to an expensive drug for treating a serious vision problem breached European Union competition rules, the EU Court of Justice ruled, and this ruling upheld a 2014 decision by Italy's antitrust authority that the drug makers colluded to boost sales of Lucentis by discrediting the cheaper Avastin drug by emphasizing potential side effects.[11] Finally, in 2014, the Japanese

Health Ministry filed a criminal complaint against the pharmaceutical company Novartis, calling for an investigation into the drug company's local unit. It is suspected that falsified data were used in the clinical trial of Novartis's best-selling drug Diovan.[12] This is most definitely a worldwide issue.

The types of fraud run the gamut of almost everything you can think of (figure 23). We tend to think that pharmaceutical cheating is reserved for off-label promotion practices. But it's not. From concealing study data to overcharging government health programs, these transgressions are indiscriminate.

And when we talk about twenty-five years of settlements and court judgments against the pharmaceutical industry, do not forget about the big one. Opioids. There is ample evidence from unsealed court proceedings and publicly available information that drug manufacturers of opioids and drug distributors engaged in a myriad of schemes that advanced the use of opioids in America. And since none of these settlements and court judgments

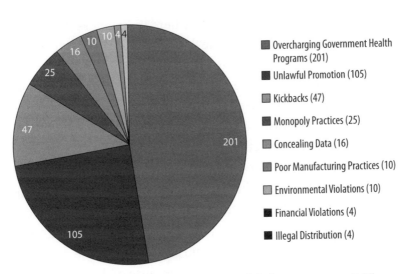

Figure 23. Types of pharmaceutical industry violations, 1991–2015. Public Citizen, *Twenty-Five Years of Pharmaceutical Industry Criminal and Civil Penalties: 1991–2015,* www.citizen.org/hrg2311.

were final in 2015, they would not be included in any statistics. In early 2020, it was reported that three giant drug distributors—McKesson, AmerisourceBergen, and Cardinal Health—were negotiating a deal with the states to end thousands of opioid lawsuits nationwide, in which they would pay $19.2 billion over eighteen years and immediately submit to stringent oversight and regulation to ensure that suspicious orders for prescription opioids would be discontinued since they had turned a blind eye to the problem by shipping more than sixty billion opioid pills across the country between 2006 and 2014.[13] This proposed settlement says nothing of the potential financial restitution that the actual drug manufacturers are negotiating with states, cities, and counties in America. We know that Purdue Pharma, the maker of OxyContin, made an offer of $10 billion. Teva and Johnson and Johnson have also been negotiating a settlement as part of a larger bundled financial deal rumored to be north of the Purdue number.[14]

It doesn't seem as though there are any lasting ramifications, however, for any corporate malfeasance. Pay a fine and move on. Unlike provider or patient fraud, where there are real jail sentences and repercussions, or the data breaches that cost companies actual money to deploy for upgrades and investments in cybersecurity, these corporate violations hit the front pages and then vanish into thin air. We need to care a little more, no? Forget about the fact that the industry continues to erode the public trust. With an alarmingly low reputation among consumers to begin with, forget about the destruction of the positive net social benefit to society every time a manufacturer engages in fraudulent behavior of any kind. Forget about the fact that making lifesaving medicines is no good if you rob the public purse or falsify and distort data. We need to care because fraud costs lives. People are dying or living with unnecessary morbidity because of these actions.

From a behavioral perspective, remedy for health care fraud seems like a simple discussion. The financial penalties imposed are not strict or severe enough to modify the behavior. Increase the fines, right? Make these companies pay more and more until they get it. Unfortunately, that may not work either. Let's just agree that a quarter of a century of data from groups such as Public Citizen doesn't seem to support the idea that financial penalties will stop this behavior. What if we impose heftier fines? Companies then have to lay off workers or make hard decisions about investing in new plants and equipment to make other medicines that had nothing to do with the original transgression. Or cut back on their research and development spending for the next few years to help defray the cost of a multi-billion-dollar court settlement. It is complicated.

So, what will change the behavior? Jail time for executives has not been a disincentive. Public shaming has not stemmed the tide of bad behavior. Maybe we should knock some time off the patent life of the molecule? But this is problematic. What do we do with generic culprits where there is no patent to deal with? Even if we're dealing with an innovator manufacturer, what if the loss of sales from a truncated patent life is less than the financial penalty? Other ideas have been floated as well. But none seem to have gained any traction. The reality is that this continues to happen precisely because imposing any sort of meaningful penalty that will change behavior is difficult to do. And the industry knows that. These transgressions are not accidents. Hiding clinical trial data doesn't just happen. Providing kickbacks and promoting products off-label requires concerted effort on behalf of many actors. Can we look to other industries for a solution? It does not appear so, as Google, Apple, and Volkswagen continue to merrily skip along after paying their respective fines.

It's a pervasive and systemic societal problem. As one senior executive in the industry told me, "If nothing changes, this will continue to happen." When pressed for a rationale, he said "because for us, it's only money."

What I have discussed in this chapter so far is what can be termed *conventional fraud*. But there is a new, alarming frontier in the health care fraud landscape. In 2019 an obviously doctored video of US Speaker of the House Nancy Pelosi appeared online. The video attempted to show her in a less-than-flattering light by slowing down her voice to give the impression that she was impaired, incoherent, or possibly inebriated. Some people found it funny. Some people were outraged. Almost contemporaneously, information that discouraged people to get their children vaccinated had gone viral on social media platforms and may have contributed to the 2019 surge in the measles outbreak in the United States.

When questioned on CNN about the Nancy Pelosi video, Facebook Vice President for Product Policy and Counterterrorism Monika Bickert stated that viewers and users are "being alerted that this video is false."[15] That's a nice soundbite. But it's hollow. Providing someone with a message that the content they are viewing or reading has been flagged and directing them to fact-checking links is a dubious strategy at best. At a behavioral level, this requires the user to do some work on their own. At a practical level, in a time-constrained world, this rarely happens with any degree of critical mass.

In response to the anti-vaccine content, Facebook said, "It is exploring additional measures to best combat the problem." That might include "reducing or removing this type of content from recommendations, including *Groups You Should Join*, and demoting it in search results, while also ensuring that higher quality and more authoritative information is available."[16]

Bickert went on to affirm that Facebook's policy is to work with independent fact-checking organizations who drive the decisions about fake versus real content and that Facebook does not make these decisions. While this is a necessary check and balance on the system, it only works if you address the fake content quickly and remove it. It does not work if you take days to verify your fact-checkers' claims and then decide that you're going to keep the content online but flag it for viewers, a toothless end run around the issue. In reality, lawmakers and, indeed, everyday people like you and me have concluded that Facebook, and other social media platforms like it, are selective, inconsistent, and ambivalent about clamping down on this misinformation. We need look no further than the assessment of current and ex-employees of these social media companies who routinely challenge chief executives about the role these platforms play in amplifying misinformation and disinformation, ranging from systemic racism to QAnon to vaccine efficacy.

Here's the rub: if social media platforms continue to establish rules of engagement that do not include the truthful and accurate reporting or posting of content, then it's just a matter of time before this problem becomes more widespread, and it may already be too late. I have advocated long and hard about the potential impact of inaccurate and deceptive online health care information. The fact that patients have difficulty distinguishing between high and low value health care information. And how high health literacy is strongly associated with better health outcomes as compared to low health literacy. And how we need to have a better system to adjudicate, authenticate, and validate online health information.

These recent and ongoing examples of shameless deceit paint an increasingly urgent picture of the current state of online misinformation, obfuscation, and misdirection. With their staggering reach, social media platforms and search engines have been weaponized to deliver false information. This misinformation is not an isolated or innocuous case of some lunatic fringe group or lone wolf individual that posts a single, benign piece of content in the far-flung corners of the dark web.

For health care, this dangerous trend of questionable information has implications that touch on all aspects of our industry. And this is problematic. Because today it is about vaccinations and the impact on measles or COVID-19. Tomorrow it may be about adverse events for a particular drug therapy that potentially drives people to avoid complying with their medication. Next week, it is about a fake post showing that Indian and Chinese manufacturers are using dangerous active pharmaceutical ingredients to manufacture drug therapies. And the week after, this misinformation is about a local hospital's emergency room being overcrowded so that patients are directed elsewhere. And in an election year, it is about a presidential candidate's health status (see Hillary Clinton circa 2016).[17] And with a raging pandemic that can circumnavigate the globe in a matter of weeks, infecting tens of millions of people, it is about whether you should wear a mask, wash your hands, and social distance. Or whether taking hydroxychloroquine is helpful and whether staying away from mass gatherings makes a difference in preventing the spread of an airborne, respiratory virus.

The solution is not obvious. And even if it were, it would be tremendously complicated. But health care is in the crosshairs of this growing and disturbing trend of deepfake content, obfuscation, misdirection, and deceitful propagation of information.

We must, collectively, lead the way on this issue. This does not mean trying to control every piece of content on the internet or to correct every snippet of misinformation. But it does mean that we must act with urgency. It means that we cannot rely on these massive social media conglomerates to fix the issue themselves in a silo. This may be an opportunity to demonstrate what has always been true of health care from any perspective: it is always about the patients. If this is true, then this issue must be one that we prioritize and address immediately. Because the people who suffer the most are the patients. While some will tell you—insist, in fact—that social media should not be arbiters of truth and that we must adhere to the fundamental proposition of freedom of speech, remember that health care's dalliances with freedom of speech are long and well documented.

18

Let Freedom Ring

For to be free is not merely to cast off one's chains, but to live in a way that respects and enhances the freedom of others.

—NELSON ROLIHLAHLA MANDELA

We are a curious bunch, are we not? Incredibly passionate about our civil liberties and the right to freely express our beliefs. But sometimes this freedom of expression conflicts with other things that are important, such as our health.

For years, the pharmaceutical industry and its lobbyists have been advocating for the unimpeded flow of information to physicians citing the US Constitution's First Amendment as the basis for their thinking. The First Amendment states that "Congress shall make no law respecting an establishment of religion, or prohibiting the free exercise thereof; or abridging the freedom of speech, or of the press; or the right of the people peaceably to assemble, and to petition the government for a redress of grievances."[1] Pretty heavy stuff, no? As Kim and Kapczynski wrote in their 2017 paper:

Since 1962, the US Food and Drug Administration (FDA) has required companies to establish, with adequate and well-controlled clinical trials, a drug's safety and efficacy for each intended use and has prohibited the "off-label" promotion of drugs. For companies to market an approved medicine for new indications, they must first conduct trials and submit data to establish safety and efficacy, as was the case for the initial approval. The FDA's approach to off-label promotion is in jeopardy, however. In response to recent US Supreme Court decisions strengthening First Amendment protection for companies, the pharmaceutical industry has framed off-label marketing as a free speech right. Drug companies have won several important court cases that have weakened the FDA's authority to regulate off-label marketing.[2]

How did the industry end up in the position where the First Amendment and freedom of speech are used as a shield to allow pharmaceutical companies to knowingly disseminate information about their molecules where the long-term safety, tolerability, and efficacy data for an unapproved indication is, at best, unclear? How did we end up with well-heeled lobbyists on Capitol Hill beating the drum vociferously to allow drug representatives to suggest that Topamax, which is approved to treat seizures and migraine head-aches, might be used in alcohol dependency or that Neurontin, which is approved for epilepsy, might be helpful in bipolar disorder or insomnia?[3] We ended up in this position partly because of the landmark *United States v. Caronia* case. Alfred Caronia was a pharmaceutical sales representative for Orphan Medical who, together with a physician in Orphan's speaker program, promoted the drug Xyrem for off-label uses. After a trial, Caronia was convicted under specific sections of the Federal Food, Drug, and Cosmetic Act. But then the Second Circuit Court of Appeals overturned

Caronia's conviction, citing his First Amendment rights. It declared that the government could not prosecute a pharmaceutical sales representative simply for making off-label promotional statements but was also careful not to entirely strike down the FDA's authority to regulate off-label promotion. *United States v. Caronia* is one of the landmark cases in this ongoing battle between the industry, the regulators, and the government that has shed light on off-label promotion. Another monumental case *Amarin Pharma, Inc. v. FDA*, which was rendered when a US District Court handed down a ruling "that the US Food and Drug Administration (FDA) lacked the authority to prohibit non-misleading forms of off-label speech."[4] It is not as though we are all neophytes and prudes. We all know that off-label promotion happens and that, more important, with or without the promotion, that off-label usage happens. Off-label drug use (i.e., prescribing medications for a different disease or medical condition, different route of administration, and/or different dosage than that approved by the FDA) is relatively common. A 2006 study estimated that 21 percent of commonly used drugs are prescribed off-label.[5] Despite the regular and sometimes medically necessary off-label use of prescription drugs (including significant utilization in certain disease states such as pediatrics, cancer, and psychotic disorders), manufacturers are only allowed to promote their products for the indication approved on the label—at least this was the prevailing view pre-*Caronia* and pre-*Amarin*.[6]

Aside from the constitutional arguments allowing for the truthful promotion of off-label information, other rationales have been floated, too. The argument that time-consuming and expensive clinical trials for every indication serve no one's best interest because of delays in making potential useful therapies available is fair. The argument that social media and sophisticated platforms make data overwhelmingly easy to access and render drug labels out of touch with real-world practice is also fair. The argument that clinicians rely on manufacturers who know more about the molecules they promote than anyone for up-to-date and relevant information is acceptable.

The other arguments are also just as persuasive, however. That the FDA serves a purpose by requiring rigorous trials to validate a drug's safety and efficacy and that circumventing this would put us on a very slippery slope. That an individual or company with much to gain financially by promoting the off-label use of its drug is in a conflict-of-interest position and should not be in a position to unilaterally decide what information can and cannot be made available. That we need to distinguish between active off-label promotion and unsolicited off-label requests from clinicians because somewhere and somehow the information that helps advance treatment needs to be shared. And this should not be a point that is glossed over. These are two fundamental, but critical, distinctions. If a manufacturer is hiring a sales force and arming them with the training to go out and flaunt the off-label usage of a drug for an indication in which a handful of case reports can be found in the public literature, versus handling a few dozen solicited requests from clinicians about whether there is any data for the use of drug X in condition Y, that is an apples and oranges scenario. It is the former that is of concern and for which massive investigations and Department of Justice fines have been levied against pharmaceutical companies.

Have we taken the freedom of speech argument too far? Are we comfortable with leading the charge for drugs to be used in patient populations for which there is no indication and, more important, no definitive body of evidence touting their safe use? Is it up to the industry to fight this battle? Or are the current regulations around off-label promotion so antiquated, restrictive, and overprotective that some coordinated effort is necessary? There is no debate that the off-label utilization of drug molecules in unapproved indications takes place and, in many instances, gets published or presented at the podium. The question is, Who decides what should be shared and who should actually do the sharing? Some have argued for a new paradigm, suggesting that all parties involved should

> work toward establishing a clear and codified "safe harbor" process (through new legislation that also will harmonize the existing FDA patchwork of off-label guidance) to prereview, amend, and qualify off-label communication to ensure that it is non-misleading. By developing such a system, manufacturers would be incentivized to both presubmit and collaboratively work with the agency to formulate off-label communication that is evidence based, is of benefit to clinicians and their patients, and could also mitigate adversarial legal proceedings between industry and the FDA.[7]

On its face, the idea is sound. In practical terms, I doubt whether this will work. This process would need to be mandatory, not voluntary. The FDA would need resources to address prereview documents and data in a timely manner. And there would have to be some sort of mediation or arbitration process to deal with disputes.

The unfortunate part of this debate is that it seems to have turned into a constitutional argument about what ought to be allowable speech as a matter of principle. We seem to have forgotten that the purpose of off-label promotion and utilization of drugs has always been to help patients who have exhausted all other treatment options. The role of an off-label medication is, after all, not as a first-line treatment option. So, if these are really sick patients for whom nothing else has worked, do we want to stop them from having access to a therapy that might provide meaningful benefit?

The other unfortunate outcome of the *Amarin* decision is that it potentially

> invites a world where companies no longer pursue broad clinical indications for new drugs but instead seek the narrowest possible

indication for approval and then market the drug for any new use for which there is some evidence, no matter how weak. Companies would no longer have to conduct rigorous trials and submit, to the FDA, data demonstrating the safety and efficacy of new uses. Such an approach would compromise the future evidence base for medicines, expose patients to a greater risk of adverse events, and increase pharmaceutical spending without evidence that the expenditures would help improve patients' health.[8]

The conversation is now about how manufacturers should be able to have a louder voice and a greater role in disseminating off-label information. Instead, what's important is the mechanism by which we get information to clinicians so that they can make treatment decisions that advance care for patients. If that means that industry is removed from the process and we leave clinicians to get this information on their own with some degree of modified or restructured regulatory oversight, then so be it.

At the center of the entire off-label promotion story is the doctor. At the end of the day, off-label promotion is directed at the doctor, who has a patient in mind for an unapproved use of a drug. But what happens when we have medications approved for a certain use and patients who want to use the medication for its approved indication, but the doctor simply refuses to prescribe it. There is no off-label usage required. No Supreme Court decision to read. No transgression of any FDA-approved label. A drug is available. A patient needs it. A doctor refuses. Or, to take it a step further, a drug is available but a doctor refuses to see the patient, completely ignoring the need and underlying diagnosis. At the extreme, the drug's availability is irrelevant, as is its need and both are afterthoughts because the doctor simply refuses to see the patient period. Is this an act of freedom of expression?

There was an uproar in Canada some years ago over the case of a young woman who visited a walk-in clinic to get her birth control prescription renewed and was refused by the physician on duty on the grounds that he didn't believe in contraception because it conflicted with his religious and/or moral beliefs.[9] And there are numerous other examples of similar scenarios from all over the world. Unlike the freedom of speech argument used by drug companies and countered by the FDA for the off-label promotion of drugs, this act of freedom of expression is initiated by the doctor who is no longer an innocent bystander on the receiving end of off-label information.

An op-ed piece in Canada's national newspaper at the time sought to frame the issue not as an attempt by a clinician to force his religious beliefs on a patient but, rather, as a larger debate on whether it is indeed possible or desirable to remove conscience from the practice of medicine. The list of treatments on which a clinician can impose his or her moral view and for which there can be legitimate conscientious objection are long: contraception, abortion, blood transfusion, cannabis use, and organ retrieval and donation—to name a few.

That there is no right or wrong is abundantly clear. It is difficult to compartmentalize one's strongly held beliefs or check them at the door by virtue of throwing on some scrubs or putting on a lab coat and stethoscope. Pillars of the community, from all walks of life, and with the highest educations have been roasted on Twitter and Instagram for comments and opinions that are racist, degrading, and insensitive. One's profession does not provide some invisible force field against bad judgment and abhorrent thoughts. Yet does the denial of a prescription for birth control fall into that category? It depends on who you ask. Let's be clear, if there is a contraindication to the treatment or a patient safety issue of some sort, there really is no argument. Everyone would agree that the clinical judgment of the doctor along with best practice guidelines and current standard of care would dictate the actions, and there would be very little uproar. In this Canadian case of the young woman who was refused oral contraception, however, the doctor did not cite the long-term deleterious effects of prolonged oral contraceptive use as his rationale for denying the renewal. He just simply refused on moral ground.

The other simmering issue in this Canadian case is that this was a prescription *renewal* and not an initial visit with patient counseling, a better and complete understanding of the patient's lifestyle and behavior or any sort of clinical workup. Another peer and colleague of this clinician somewhere else in the city had already determined that oral contraceptives were both safe and appropriate to prescribe for this patient (i.e., they fit the construct of the original doctor's moral beliefs and clinical judgment). So, this doctor actually reversed the clinical decision making of a peer by denying the renewal of the prescription.

The typical knee-jerk reaction in situations like this is to suggest that health care is different and that medicine is special, so we can't compare this denial of oral contraception to other scenarios involving civil liberties such as freedom of speech and freedom of expression. We've conditioned ourselves to believe that when we're talking about health care there are no rules and everything is an exception. An incredible echo chamber reverberates in health care. If your Jewish airline pilot refused to fly through Arab airspace on moral grounds, would this be acceptable? Would we suggest that it is not necessarily possible or desirable to remove conscience from the airline industry or that a system without conscience is not in the best interests of consumers? If a waitress refused to serve you beef on the moral ground that she is Hindu and does not believe in the slaughter of cows for human consumption, what would we say?

This op-ed piece from many years ago went on to suggest that "in this wonderfully diverse [Canada] country with its diverse cultures and beliefs, we can tolerate a little diversity among physicians." But that has nothing to do with the situation and Canada might as well be a proxy for any number of countries that have the same richly diverse cultural fabric. Diversity among physicians certainly has a place in any society, but the question is, Where does the diversity start, and where does it end? Is refusing to provide someone with a medication because of one's moral beliefs diversity? Some would argue it is not. Who interprets what constitutes diversity anyway? Policy folks? Lawmakers? Politicians? Clinicians? This is a slippery slope. The College of Physicians and Surgeons issued a statement endorsed by a Catholic archbishop, a rabbi, and an imam and it read as follows: "No Canadian citizen, including any physician, should ever be disciplined or risk losing their professional standing for conducting their work in the conformity with their most deeply held ethical or religious convictions." The only problem with this statement is that they forgot this imaginary last line: *unless it conflicts with and impinges upon the most deeply held ethical, moral, or religious convictions of their patients.*

In November 2019, a federal judge overturned the Trump administration's attempt to expand the conscience rule, which was "aimed at protecting doctors, nurses, and others from, in the words of the United States Department of Health and Human Services, being 'bullied out of the health care field' for refusing to participate in abortions, gender reassignment surgery, or other medical procedures based on religious beliefs or conscience."[10] To be fair, there are definitive conditions that experts have outlined in which it is deemed acceptable for physicians to withhold care and services. Sarah C. Hull, one of those experts and a cardiologist at Yale School of Medicine and associate director of its Program for Biomedical Ethics, suggests that there are three conditions under which physicians can withhold care: "when doctors are subjected to abusive treatment, when the treatment requested is outside a doctor's scope of practice, or when providing the requested treatment would otherwise violate one's duties as a physician, such as the Hippocratic mandate to 'first do no harm.'" Outside of these specific scenarios, Hull writes,

> it is not a physician's job to tell patients how to live according to the physician's personal code of ethics, whether religious or secular. Nor should a physician withhold treatment from patients simply because they fail to adhere to his or her personal standards of morality. Rather, a physician's duty is to promote patients' wellness and flourishing through the application of evidence-based medicine to the best of his or her professional ability. Personal beliefs, religious or otherwise, must not interfere with that. There is nothing conscientious about doctors objecting to caring for patients when we simply disagree with how our patients live their lives. It is unethical for doctors to bully patients in the name of our personal convictions—a blatant violation of our professional duty. We owe it to ourselves and to our patients to hold our profession to a higher standard.[11]

Hull is careful, of course, to discuss the conflict presented with abortion and physician-assisted suicide and notes that in these conditions, there is some legitimate concern that conscientious objection not be overlooked.

In the end, the freedom to believe, to speak, and to act cuts many ways in health care. The overriding perspective that I have always taken is that, if the patient is at the center of our desire to enforce these freedoms, then we are headed in the right direction. But, as this chapter shows, that is not always the case. Sometimes we need to defend the industry's right to deliver non-misleading information or a doctor's right to take a stand on a moral issue. The realization that the patient is not first in the conversation is jarring. But sometimes everyone needs to give a little, so that everyone wins a little.

Conclusion

Predicting rain doesn't count. Building arks does.

—WARREN BUFFETT, Noah Rule

Warren Buffett's quote appeared in a 2001 Berkshire Hathaway shareholder report to explain the big mistake he made that year. In Buffett's estimation, Berkshire Hathaway had a terrible year, and the impact was compounded by the tragic events of September 11, 2001. Buffett was explaining that he had actually predicted many of the market events that happened *before* that fateful day, but he "didn't convert thought to action," thus violating the Noah Rule (the rain came as he expected, but he hadn't built an ark).[1]

The cynical reader might scoff at the attribution of some fancy moniker to what we all know simply as planning ahead. Or what some call planning two steps ahead.

In case A happens, I should plan to do B. Duh.

What makes most really smart, successful people really smart and successful is that they actually plan for B (it's not some ethereal concept that they aspire to achieve one day in the future) and that they use the power of experience and knowledge to guide their decisions. Most people can predict rain both literally and figuratively. Let's take the literal scenario: I can look at the sky, search for some Doppler radar to show the movement of the rain clouds, and then check my phone's Weather Channel app. After doing these things, I'll have some reasonably accurate prediction of the likelihood of rain. But then comes the tricky part. The converting-thought-to-action part. I need to turn off the sprinklers, cover the cushions on the deck chairs, and make sure the roof of my convertible parked in the driveway is closed. If I do those things, I have just built an ark.

The essence of the Noah Rule is that we ought to imbue some sort of Bayesian practicality into how we think, plan, and execute anything and everything. Bayes' theorem—or at least its basic precept—is that the probability of an event occurring is based on prior knowledge of variables and factors related to that event. In real-world terms, the probability that I will make all the red lights on the way to drop my kids off at school and get them there on time is a function of what day of the week it is, the time I leave my house, and the route I actually take. I know this because I have done it hundreds of times. In other words, I am using my prior knowledge of factors and variables related to dropping my kids off at school to help me understand the probability of making these red lights.

Simple, yes?

But nothing in health care is simple. This is why the Noah Rule is one of the unmistakable takeaways from my book. It's not enough to know it's going to rain; we have to get down to the business of building arks. Do we really need to predict that drug companies are going to charge a lot for new medications? Let's plan to do something about it based on our knowledge of prior events related to drug pricing. When they do, we're ready. If they don't, no harm done. Let's stop only *predicting* whether some misinformation or disinformation is going to strangle epidemiology and public health's ability to effect and galvanize change as more dangerous zoonotic viruses appear, and let's assume it's going to happen based on what we know and have learned about anti-vaxxers, the COVID-19 pandemic, and social media misinformation in the twenty-first century. Let's build an ark for that right now. If it happens (which is likely), we're ready. If it doesn't happen, it doesn't happen. Either way, we've got the ark built for that scenario. Let's stop guessing which social determinant of health has a bigger effect on access to health care during the next global pandemic. We already know that communities of color are disproportionately affected. We know that communities suffering from housing insecurity are at extremely high risk. We know that people who don't have white-collar jobs tailor made for social distancing because they can hop on Zoom calls all day are exposed and vulnerable. Let's just get after it and fix it. Build the ark. Appropriate the congressional funding. Get the private sector involved. Whatever, as long as we're taking action in meaningful ways.

For too long, we have been great at predicting what can and will happen in health care. But we have failed miserably at building the ark. We have surrounded ourselves with sacred cows and cocooned ourselves in obvious echo chambers. The solutions to health care's biggest problems are more than a planning issue. We need disciples committed to the cause. We need money. We need political will. We need luck, patience, and hard work. We need to be bold and take risks.

Most of all, we need to learn to live with the rain.

ACKNOWLEDGMENTS

There is a parable that I read when I was much younger, where an ad in a magazine was seeking a new sportswriter for the local paper. Interested applicants were asked to come down and apply in person with the editor of the sports department. A young man saw the ad and hurried down to the newspaper's offices and excitedly announced that he wanted to see the sports editor so that he could apply for the job. The sports editor called him into his office and asked him, "So, what makes you think you're my next sportswriter?" The young applicant replied confidently, "Well, it's very simple sir, I love sports." The editor got up from his desk and walked over to the young man and placed a gentle hand on his shoulder and said to him "Son, come back when you love writing."

It is difficult to write a book. Many days are frustrating, and the ideas just don't seem to flow. Distractions get in the way. Writer's block is a real thing. But the love of writing cannot be quelled for it, too, is a real thing.

At the end of a journey like this, there are so many people to acknowledge. I want to start by thanking Martha Murphy who answered my LinkedIn request back in the summer of 2016 and agreed to work with me. She helped shape my book proposal and provided much needed guidance to a neophyte author such as myself. I also want to thank Robin W. Coleman, my acquisitions editor at Johns Hopkins University Press, for showing interest in my proposal. Working with Robin to develop the manuscript was a tremendous experience and his thoughtful approach to the book, its audience, and the subject matter allowed me to develop a book of which I am exceptionally proud. I also want to thank the entire JHUP team for their unwavering support and encouragement in helping to shepherd this book across the finish line. I want to thank the countless physicians, patients, classmates, and professors who I have interacted with over the years and who have imbued within me a global perspective about health care and, more importantly, a balanced one.

But most of all I want to thank my family. My wife and two daughters have been unfailingly supportive and encouraging in this endeavor. They have borne witness to the early mornings and the incessant pleas for "quiet time" so that I could finish a thought or a sentence or a page. This book is their book, too. And specifically for my daughters, there is an important lesson in this book. That ideas matter. That effort matters. And belief matters. And finishing what you start matters. And setting lofty goals matters. May this book remind them of these things throughout their lives.

NOTES

Chapter 1. All the King's Men

1. Gerald F. Anderson et al., "It's the Prices, Stupid: Why the United States Is So Different from Other Countries," *Health Affairs* 22, no. 3 (May/June 2003): 89–105.

2. "Wikipedia: Martin Shkreli," Wikimedia Foundation, last modified November 22, 2020, 02:55, https://en.wikipedia.org/wiki/Martin_Shkreli.

3. Anna Almendrala, "What the Darprim Price Hike Actually Does to Health Care," *HUFFPOST*, September 23, 2015, https://www.huffingtonpost.ca/entry/daraprim-price-turing-shkreli_us_560063cee4b00310edf82060.

4. Robert Langreth and Drew Armstrong, "Clinton's Tweet on High Drug Prices Sends Biotech Stocks Down," Bloomberg, September 21, 2015, https://www.bloomberg.com/news/articles/2015-09-21/clinton-s-tweet-on-high-drug-prices-sends-biotech-stocks-down.

5. Malcolm Gladwell, *The Tipping Point: How Little Things Can Make a Big Difference* (Boston: Little, Brown, 2000).

6. "Mylan CEO on EpiPen Drug Price Controversy: 'I Get the Outrage,'" *CBS News*, https://www.cbsnews.com/news/epipen-price-hike-controversy-mylan-ceo-heather-bresch-speaks-out/.

7. "What Is an EpiPen and Who Needs It?," Atlanta Allergy & Asthma, updated November 9, 2020, https://www.atlantaallergy.com/posts/view/33-what-is-an-epipen-and-who-needs-it.

8. Jonathan D. Rockoff, "Mylan Faces Scrutiny over EpiPen Price Increases," *Wall Street Journal*, April 21, 2016, https://www.wsj.com/articles/mylan-faces-scrutiny-over-epipen-price-increases-1472074823.

9. "Full Prescribing Information," RESTASIS, Allergan, revised July 2017, https://www.allergan.com/assets/pdf/restasis_pi.pdf.

10. "Prescriber Checkup," RESTASIS, ProPublica, https://projects.propublica.org/checkup/drugs/5331.

11. Lisa M. Schwartz and Steven Woloshin, "A Clear-Eyed View of Restasis and Chronic Dry Eye Disease," *JAMA Internal Medicine* 178, no. 2 (2018): 181–182.

12. Dartmouth College, "Restasis: Why US Consumers Paid Billions for Drug Deemed Ineffective in Other Countries," Medical Xpress, January 2, 2018, https://medicalxpress.com/news/2018-01-restasis-consumers-paid-billions-drug.html

13. Lydia Ramsey Pflanzer, "One of Allergan's Blockbuster Drugs Was Dealt a Major Legal Blow," *Business Insider*, October 15, 2017, https://www .businessinsider.com/allergan-restasis-patents-invalid-in-texas-district -court-2017-10.

14. "Our Social Contract with Patients," Allergan, September 6, 2016, https://allergan-web-us-prod.azurewebsites.net/news/ceo-blog/september -2016/our-social-contract-with-patients.

15. "Our Social Contract with Patients."

16. M. M. Denniston et al., "Chronic Hepatitis C Virus Infection in the United States, National Health and Nutrition Examination Survey 2003 to 2010," *Annals of Internal Medicine* 160, no. 5 (2014): 293–300.

17. Centers for Disease Control and Prevention, "Viral Hepatitis: Q&As for the Public," CDC, October 17, 2016, www.cdc.gov/hepatitis/hcv/cfaq .htm#cFAQ22.

18. John Rother, "What I Learned at the Brookings Institution," National Coalition on Health Care, October 1, 2014, https://nchc.org/what-i-learned -at-the-brookings-institution/.

19. Jane Horvath, "Legal Challenges for Rx Drug Laws Passed in 2017 Will Shape Future States' Cost Containment Legislation," National Academy for State Health Policy, March 2018, https://nashp.org/wp-content /uploads/2018/03/Legal-States-on-Rx-Law.pdf.

20. Makiko Kitamura and Johannes Koch, "When Cancer Treatments Fail, Italy Wants Money Back," Bloomberg, January 15, 2016, corrected April 19, 2016, http://www.bloomberg.com/news/articles/2016-01-15/when -new-cancer-treatments-fail-italy-wants-its-money-back.

21. Himanshu Gupta et al., "Patent Protection Strategies," *Journal of Pharmacy and Bioallied Sciences* 2, no. 1 (2010): 2.

Chapter 2. Heads I Win, Tails You Lose

1. Daniel Kahneman and Amos Tversky, "Prospect Theory: An Analysis of Decision under Risk," *Econometrica* 47, no. 2 (1984): 263–292; Kahneman and Tversky, "Choices, Values, and Frames," *American Psychologist* 39 (1979): 341–350.

2. From Dan Ariely's TED Talk, "Are We in Control of Our Own Decisions?," 2008, https://www.ted.com/talks/dan_ariely_are_we_in_control _of_our_own_decisions?language=en.

3. This analysis is from the Economist/YouGov Poll conducted by YouGov/Polimetrix. The survey of one thousand respondents was conducted August 23–25, 2009.

4. David L. Eckles and Brian F. Schaffner, "Loss Aversion and the Framing of the Health Care Reform Debate," *The Forum* 8, no. 1 (2010).

Chapter 3. The UnHappiness Project

1. Ryan T. Howell, Margaret L. Kern, and Sonja Lyubomirsky, "Health Benefits: Meta-analytically Determining the Impact of Well-Being on Objective Health Outcomes," *Health Psychology Review* 1, no. 1 (2007): 83–136.

2. Carol Graham, "Happiness and Health: Lessons—and Questions—for Public Policy," *Health Affairs (Millwood)* 27, no. 1 (2008): 72–87.

3. Justin McCarthy, "Big Pharma Sinks to the Bottom of U.S. Industry Rankings," Gallup, September 3, 2018, https://news.gallup.com/poll/266060/big-pharma-sinks-bottom-industry-rankings.aspx?.

4. Theo Vos et al., "Global, Regional, and National Incidence, Prevalence, and Years Lived with Disability for 301 Acute and Chronic Diseases and Injuries in 188 Countries, 1990–2013: A Systematic Analysis for the Global Burden of Disease Study 2013," *The Lancet* 386, no. 9995 (2015): 743–800.

5. Kok Fong See and Siew Hwa Yen, "Does Happiness Matter to Health System Efficiency? A Performance Analysis," *Health Economics Review* 8, no. 1 (2018): 33.

6. "About the GSS," General Social Survey, NORC, 2016, https://gss.norc.org/About-The-GSS.

7. Richard A. Easterlin, "Explaining Happiness," *Proceedings of the National Academy of Sciences* 100, no. 19 (2003): 11176–11783.

8. Easterlin, "Explaining Happiness."

9. J. Helliwell, R. Layard, and J. Sachs, *World Happiness Report 2017* (New York: Sustainable Development Solutions Network, 2017).

10. World Health Organization, "Preamble to the Constitution of the World Health Organization as adopted by the International Health Conference" (New York, June 19–22, 1946); signed on July 22, 1946, by the representatives of 61 States (Official Records of the World Health Organization, no. 2, p. 100) and entered into force on April 7, 1948, http://www.who.int/governance/eb/who_constitution_en.pdf (1948).

11. Rodolfo Saracci, "The World Health Organisation Needs to Reconsider Its Definition of Health," *BMJ* 314, no. 7091 (1997): 1409–1410.

Chapter 4. Customer Satisfaction

1. Janet Adamy, "US Ties Hospital Payments to Making Patients Happy," *WSJ Online*, October 14, 2012.

2. Owen Bowcott, "Hospital Funding to Be Based on Patient Satisfaction," *The Guardian*, December 10, 2009, https://www.theguardian.com/society/2009/dec/10/hospital-funds-based-patient-satisfaction.

3. *Ontario's Action Plan for Health Care* (Toronto: Queen's Printer for Ontario, 2012), http://www.health.gov.on.ca/en/ms/ecfa/healthy_change/docs/rep_healthychange.pdf.

4. Adamy, "US Ties Hospital Payments to Making Patients Happy."

5. "Patient Experience in Canadian Hospitals," CIHI, 2019, https://www.cihi.ca/en/patient-experience/patient-experience-in-canadian-hospitals.

6. John Sitzia, "How Valid and Reliable Are Patient Satisfaction Data? An Analysis of 195 Studies," *International Journal for Quality in Health Care* 11, no. 4 (1999): 319–328.

7. W. Boulding et al., "Relationship between Patient Satisfaction with Inpatient Care and Hospital Readmission within 30 Days," *American Journal of Managed Care* 17 (2011): 41–48.

8. Boulding et al., "Relationship between Patient Satisfaction."

9. Matthew P. Manary et al., "The Patient Experience and Health Outcomes," *New England Journal of Medicine* 368, no. 3 (2013): 201–203.

10. Manary et al., "The Patient Experience."

11. Joshua J. Fenton et al., "The Cost of Satisfaction: A National Study of Patient Satisfaction, Health Care Utilization, Expenditures, and Mortality," *Archives of Internal Medicine* 172, no. 5 (2012): 405–411.

Chapter 5. I Still Haven't Found What I'm Looking For

1. Janet M. Morahan-Martin, "How Internet Users Find, Evaluate, and Use Online Health Information: A Cross-Cultural Review," *Cyberpsychology & Behaviour* 7, no. 5 (2004): 498.

2. Jane Weaver, "More People Search for Health Online," *NBC News*, July 16, 2003, http://www.nbcnews.com/id/3077086/t/more-people-search-health-online/#.XjmeYGhKiM8.

3. Susannah Fox and Maeve Duggan, "Health Online 2013," Pew Research Center, January 14, 2013, https://www.pewresearch.org/internet/2013/01/15/health-online-2013/.

4. Noor Van Riel et al., "The Effect of Dr Google on Doctor–Patient Encounters in Primary Care: A Quantitative, Observational, Cross-Sectional Study," *BJGP Open* 1, no. 2 (2017): bjgpopen17X100833.

5. Leo Kelion, "Google Hit with Record EU Fine over Shopping Service," *BBC News*, June 27, 2017, https://www.bbc.com/news/technology-40406542.

6. G. Eysenbach et al., "Empirical Studies Assessing the Quality of Health Information for Consumers on the World Wide Web: A Systematic Review," *Journal of the American Medical Association* 287:2691–2700.

7. Lubna Daraz et al., "Can Patients Trust Online Health Information? A Meta-narrative Systematic Review Addressing the Quality of Health Information on the Internet," *Journal of General Internal Medicine* 34, no. 9 (2019): 1884–1891.

8. Deborah Charnock et al., "DISCERN: An Instrument for Judging the Quality of Written Consumer Health Information on Treatment

Choices," *Journal of Epidemiology and Community Health* 53, no. 2 (1999): 105–111.

9. S. C. Ratzan and R. M. Parker, introduction to *National Library of Medicine Current Bibliographies in Medicine: Health Literacy*, ed. C. R. Selden et al. (Bethesda, MD: National Institutes of Health, 2000), ix.

10. N. D. Berkman et al., *Health Literacy Interventions and Outcomes: An Updated Systematic Review*, Evidence Report/Technology Assessment No. 199, AHRQ Publication No. 11-E006 (Rockville, MD: Agency for Healthcare Research and Quality, March 2011).

Chapter 6. The Rating Game

1. Jeffrey Segal, "The *Right* Way to Fight Bad Online Reviews," Medscape, November 25, 2014, https://www.medscape.com/viewarticle/835077.

2. Healthcare Consumer Insight & Digital Engagement Survey, conducted by OnePoll and commissioned by Binary Fountain, 2019 Binary Fountain Inc., https://www.binaryfountain.com/resources-white-paper-ebooks/.

3. David A. Hanauer et al., "Public Awareness, Perception, and Use of Online Physician Rating Sites," *JAMA* 311, no. 7 (2014): 734–735.

4. Jeffrey Segal, "The Role of the Internet in Doctor Performance Rating," *Pain Physician* 12, no. 3 (2009): 659–664.

5. Segal, "The Role of the Internet."

6. "Legal Protections for Anonymous Speech," Digital Media Law Project, http://www.dmlp.org/legal-guide/legal-protections-anonymous-speech.

Chapter 7. The Mother of All Nudges

1. Richard H. Thaler and Cass R. Sunstein, *Nudge: Improving Decisions about Health, Wealth, and Happiness* (New York: Penguin, 2009).

2. Thaler and Sunstein, *Nudge*.

3. Thaler and Sunstein, *Nudge*.

4. Daniel Bernoulli, "Exposition of a New Theory on the Measurement of Risk," originally published in 1738, trans. Louise Sommer, *Econometrica* 22, no. 1 (1954): 22–36.

5. "Glossary of Statistical Terms," OECD, 1993, https://stats.oecd.org/glossary/detail.asp?ID=3215.

6. Kevin Roose, "Get Ready for a Vaccine Information War," *New York Times*, May 13, 2020, https://www.nytimes.com/2020/05/13/technology/coronavirus-vaccine-disinformation.html?searchResultPosition=1.

7. Leena Paakkari and Orkan Okan, "COVID-19: Health Literacy Is an Underestimated Problem," *Lancet Public Health* 5, no. 5 (2020): E249–E250.

8. Thomas Abel and David McQueen, "Critical Health Literacy and the COVID-19 Crisis," *Health Promotion International*, April 2, 2020, doi:10.1093/heapro/daaa040.

9. Karen Hao, "Nearly Half of Twitter Accounts Pushing to Reopen America May Be Bots," *MIT Technology Review*, May 21, 2020, https://www.technologyreview.com/2020/05/21/1002105/covid-bot-twitter-accounts-push-to-reopen-america/.

Chapter 8. Your Health Is about More Than Just Your Health

1. "Social Determinants of Health," World Health Organization, 2020, https://www.who.int/social_determinants/sdh_definition/en/.

2. Lauren A. Taylor et al., "Leveraging the social determinants of health: what works?," *PLoS One* 11, no. 8 (2016): e0160217, p. 16.

3. J. Mac McCullough, "Declines in Spending Despite Positive Returns on Investment: Understanding Public Health's Wrong Pocket Problem," *Frontiers in Public Health* 7 (2019): 159.

4. T. T. Brown, "Returns on Investment in California County Departments of Public Health," *American Journal of Public Health* 106, no. 8 (2016): 1477–1482, doi:10.2105/AJPH.2016.303233.

5. G. P. Mays and S. A. Smith, "Evidence Links Increases in Public Health Spending to Declines in Preventable Deaths," *Health Affairs* 30, no. 8 (2011): 1585–1593, doi:10.1377/hlthaff.2011.0196.

6. D. U. Himmelstein and S. Woolhandler, "Public Health's Falling Share of US Health Spending," *American Journal of Public Health* 106, no. 1 (2016): 56–57, doi:10.2105/AJPH.2015.302908.

7. McCullough, "Declines in Spending," 159.

8. Sandro Galea et al., "Estimated Deaths Attributable to Social Factors in the United States," *American Journal of Public Health* 101, no. 8 (2011): 1456–1465.

9. Robert Wood Johnson Foundation, Commission to Build a Healthier America, 2020, http://www.commissiononhealth.org/Charts.aspx.

10. P. Braveman and S. Egerter, *Overcoming Obstacles to Health* (Princeton, NJ: Robert Wood Johnson Foundation, 2008).

11. N. D. Berkman et al., *Health Literacy Interventions and Outcomes: An Updated Systematic Review*, Evidence Report/Technology Assessment No. 199, AHRQ Publication No. 11-E006 (Rockville, MD: Agency for Healthcare Research and Quality, March 2011).

Chapter 9. Needle in a Haystack

1. Julie Buring, "Screening or Early Disease Detection" (lecture, Harvard T.H. Chan School of Public Health, Cambridge, MA, August 2017).

2. US Preventive Services Task Force, "Screening for Prostate Cancer," Draft Recommendation Statement, April 2017, www.screeningforprostatecancer.org.

3. Buring, "Screening or Early Disease Detection."

4. Screening for Disease, Boston University School of Public Health, https://sphweb.bumc.bu.edu/otlt/MPH-Modules/EP/EP713_Screening/EP713_Screening_print.html.

5. Buring, "Screening or Early Disease Detection."

6. Screening for Disease.

7. Buring, "Screening or Early Disease Detection."

8. Buring, "Screening or Early Disease Detection."

Chapter 10. Ghost in the Machine

1. David Amerland, *Google Semantic Search: Search Engine Optimization (SEO) Techniques That Get Your Company More Traffic, Increase Brand Impact and Amplify Your Online Presence* (Indianapolis, IN: Que, 2013).

2. "Google I/O 2013: Keynote," YouTube video, 3:25:32, https://www.youtube.com/watch?v=9pmPa_KxsAM#t=1h51m10s.

3. Karen Hao, "What Is Machine Learning?," *MIT Technology Review*, November 17, 2018, https://www.technologyreview.com/2018/11/17/103781/what-is-machine-learning-we-drew-you-another-flowchart/.

4. Hao, "What Is Machine Learning?"

5. Hao, "What Is Machine Learning?"

6. Hao, "What Is Machine Learning?"

7. Vinay Prasad and Sham Mailankody, "Research and Development Spending to Bring a Single Cancer Drug to Market and Revenues after Approval," *JAMA Internal Medicine* 177, no. 11 (2017): 1569–1575.

8. Christian Willy, Edmund A. M. Neugebauer, and Heinz Gerngroß, "The Concept of Nonlinearity in Complex Systems," *European Journal of Trauma* 29, no. 1 (2003): 11–22.

9. Eric Bender, "Unpacking the Black Box in Artificial Intelligence for Medicine," *Undark*, December 4, 2019, https://undark.org/2019/12/04/black-box-artificial-intelligence/.

10. Bender, "Unpacking the Black Box."

11. David S. Watson et al., "Clinical Applications of Machine Learning Algorithms: Beyond the Black Box," *BMJ* 364 (2019): l886.

Chapter 11. The Eye of the Storm

1. Michael Lewis, *The Fifth Risk: Undoing Democracy* (London: Penguin Books, 2018).

2. Tali Sharot, "The Optimism Bias," *Current Biology* 21, no. 23 (2011): R941–R945.

3. Sharot, "The Optimism Bias."

4. Sharot, "The Optimism Bias."

5. Iain Chalmers and Robert Matthews, "What Are the Implications of Optimism Bias in Clinical Research?," *The Lancet* 367, no. 9509 (2006): 449–450.

6. Ho-Young Ahn, Jin Seong Park, and Eric Haley, "Consumers' Optimism Bias and Responses to Risk Disclosures in Direct-to-Consumer (DTC) Prescription Drug Advertising: The Moderating Role of Subjective Health Literacy," *Journal of Consumer Affairs* 48, no. 1 (2014): 175–194.

7. Ahn et al., "Consumers' Optimism Bias."

8. Ahn et al., "Consumers' Optimism Bias."

9. D. R. Strunk, H. Lopez, and R. J. DeRubeis, "Depressive Symptoms Are Associated with Unrealistic Negative Predictions of Future Life Events," *Behaviour Research and Therapy* 44 (2006): 861–882.

10. Strunk et al., "Depressive Symptoms."

11. Mary E. Wickman, Nancy Lois Ruth Anderson, and Cindy Smith Greenberg, "The Adolescent Perception of Invincibility and Its Influence on Teen Acceptance of Health Promotion Strategies," *Journal of Pediatric Nursing* 23, no. 6 (2008): 460–468.

12. Wickman et al., "Adolescent Perception of Invincibility."

13. Michael Lewis, *The Fifth Risk: Undoing Democracy*.

Chapter 12. Homesick

1. David Adam, "A Guide to R—the Pandemic's Misunderstood Metric," *Nature*, July 3, 2020, https://www.nature.com/articles/d41586-020 -02009-w.

2. Daniel Jones et al., "Impact of the COVID-19 Pandemic on the Symptomatic Diagnosis of Cancer: The View from Primary Care," *Lancet Oncology* 21, no. 6 (2020): 748–750.

3. Jones et al., "Impact of the COVID-19 Pandemic."

4. World Health Organization, "Hard Fought Gains in Immunization Coverage at Risk without Critical Health Services, Warns WHO," press release, April 23, 2020, https://www.who.int/news/item/23-04-2020-hard -fought-gains-in-immunization-coverage-at-risk-without-critical-health -services-warns-who.

5. David Waldstein, "Vaccinations Fall to Alarming Rates, C.D.C. Study Shows," *New York Times*, May 18, 2020, updated November 18, 2020, https://www.nytimes.com/2020/05/18/health/vaccinations-rates -coronavirus.html.

6. Kelsey Piper, "The Coronavirus Crisis Is Leading to an Immuniza- tion Crisis," Vox, May 23, 20202, https://www.vox.com/future-perfect /21263982/vaccinations-childhood-coronavirus-measles.

7. Jan Hoffman, "Millions of Children Are at Risk for Measles as Coronavirus Fears Halt Vaccines," *New York Times*, April 13, 2020, https:// www.nytimes.com/2020/04/13/health/coronavirus-measles-vaccines .html.

8. Fiona M. Guerra et al., "The Basic Reproduction Number (R0) of Measles: A Systematic Review," *Lancet Infectious Diseases* 17, no. 12 (2017): e420–e428.

9. Erin Brodwin, "With Covid-19 Delaying Routine Care, Chronic Disease Startups Brace for a Slew of Complications," *STAT*, April 14, 2020, https://www.statnews.com/2020/04/14/with-covid-19-delaying-routine -care-chronic-disease-startups-brace-for-a-slew-of-complications/.

10. Christina Farr, "Hospitals Could Struggle—and More Will Go Bankrupt—Until They Get Patients Back in the Door," CNBC, June 7, 2020, https://www.cnbc.com/2020/06/07/hospitals-will-struggle-until-they-get -patients-back-in-the-door.html?_source=iosappshare%7Ccom.apple.UIKit .activity.Mail.

11. Farr, "Hospitals Could Struggle."

12. Robin Bainbridge, "US Hospitals Losing around $50 Billion a Month due to Covid-19, *ITIJ*, May 4, 2020, https://www.itij.com/latest/news/us -hospitals-losing-around-50-billion-month-due-covid-19.

13. Bainbridge, "US Hospitals Losing."

14. Bainbridge, "US Hospitals Losing."

15. Sara Berg, "How COVID-19 Is Affecting Physicians of Color across the Country," AMA, April 14, 2020, https://www.ama-assn.org/delivering-care /health-equity/how-covid-19-affecting-physicians-color-across-country.

16. Kristen Hwang, "Coronavirus Could Force Private Practices to Close or Sell—Raising Costs," CalMatters, April 24, 2020, https://calmatters.org /health/2020/04/coronavirus-private-practice-doctors/.

17. Hwang, "Coronavirus Could Force Private Practices."

18. Hwang, "Coronavirus Could Force Private Practices."

19. David Cutler, "How Will COVID-19 Affect the Health Care Economy?," *JAMA Health Forum* 1, no. 4 (2020).

20. Cutler, "How Will COVID-19."

21. Bainbridge, "US Hospitals Losing."

Chapter 13. Reefer Madness

1. Eric Schlosser, "Reefer Madness," *The Atlantic*, August 1994, https:// www.theatlantic.com/magazine/archive/1994/08/reefer-madness/303476/.

2. Schlosser, "Reefer Madness."

3. Schlosser, "Reefer Madness."

4. "Quick Facts," United States Sentencing Commission, June 2020, https://www.ussc.gov/research/quick-facts/federal-offenders-prison.

5. Antonio Waldo Zuardi, "History of Cannabis as a Medicine: A Review," *Brazilian Journal of Psychiatry* 28, no. 2 (2006): 153–157.

6. Zuardi, "History of Cannabis."

7. National Academies of Sciences, Engineering, and Medicine, *The Health Effects of Cannabis and Cannabinoids: The Current State of Evidence and Recommendations for Research* (Washington, DC: National Academies Press, 2017).

8. C. Thirlwell and S. Rivas, "The Basic Background of the Cannabis Plant, the Endocannabinoid System (ECS) and Pharmacological Features," *Medical Cannabis Today* (2020).

9. David C. Radley, Stan N. Finkelstein, and Randall S. Stafford, "Off-Label Prescribing among Office-Based Physicians," *Archives of Internal Medicine* 166, no. 9 (2006): 1021–1026.

10. Radley et al., "Off-Label Prescribing."

11. Marcus A. Bachhuber et al., "Medical Cannabis Laws and Opioid Analgesic Overdose Mortality in the United States, 1999–2010," *JAMA Internal Medicine* 174, no. 10 (2014): 1668–1673.

12. Ashley C. Bradford et al., "Association between US State Medical Cannabis Laws and Opioid Prescribing in the Medicare Part D Population," *JAMA Internal Medicine* 178, no. 5 (2018): 667–672.

13. "Overdose Deaths," Centers for Disease Control and Prevention, https://www.cdc.gov/drugoverdose/data/prescribing/overdose-death-maps .html.

Chapter 14. Customer Appreciation

1. *Merriam-Webster*, s.v. "heterogeneous (adj.)," accessed December 15, 2020, https://www.merriam-webster.com/dictionary/heterogeneous.

2. Marc L. Berk and Alan C. Monheit, "The Concentration of Health Care Expenditures, Revisited," *Health Affairs* 20, no. 2 (2001): 9–18.

3. Berk and Monheit, "Concentration of Health Care Expenditures."

4. Berk and Monheit, "Concentration of Health Care Expenditures."

5. Joseph L. Dieleman et al., "US Spending on Personal Health Care and Public Health, 1996–2013," *JAMA* 316, no. 24 (2016): 2627–2646.

6. Dieleman et al., "US Spending."

7. Dieleman et al., "US Spending."

8. Matt Ford, "America's Largest Mental Hospital Is a Jail," *The Atlantic*, June 8, 2015, https://www.theatlantic.com/politics/archive/2015/06 /americas-largest-mental-hospital-is-a-jail/395012/.

Chapter 15. Under the Influence

1. Ana M. Díaz-Martín, Anne Schmitz, and María Jesús Yagüe Guillén, "Are Health e-Mavens the New Patient Influencers?," *Frontiers in Psychology* 11 (2020): 779.

2. Ye Sun, Miao Liu, and Melinda Krakow, "Health e-Mavens: Identifying Active Online Health Information Users," *Health Expectations* 19, no. 5 (2016): 1071–1083.

3. Sun et al., "Health e-Mavens."

4. Malcolm Gladwell, *The Tipping Point: How Little Things Can Make a Big Difference* (n.p.: Little, Brown, 2006).

5. Bernie Woodall, "Tiger Didn't Help Buick Sales," *Globe and Mail*, February 12, 2010, https://www.theglobeandmail.com/sports/golf/tiger-didnt-help-buick-sales/article4306913/.

6. Chris Elkins, "Celebrities Team with Big Pharma to Promote Drugs, Disease Awareness," Drugwatch, November 9, 2015, https://www.drugwatch.com/news/2015/11/09/celebrity-and-big-pharma-drug-promotion/.

7. Elkins, "Celebrities Team with Big Pharma."

8. Elkins, "Celebrities Team with Big Pharma."

9. Harlan M. Krumholz et al., "What Have We Learnt from Vioxx?," *BMJ* 334, no. 7585 (2007): 120–123.

10. Krumholz et al., "What Have We Learnt from Vioxx?"

Chapter 16. Data Dump

1. B. MacMahon and T. F. Pugh, *Epidemiology, Principles and Methods* (Boston: Little, Brown, 1970).

2. Charles H. Hennekens and Julie E. Buring, *Epidemiology in Medicine*, Vol. 515 (Boston: Little, Brown, 1987).

3. Hennekens and Buring, *Epidemiology in Medicine*.

4. Velayutham Gopikrishna, "A Report on Case Reports," *Journal of Conservative Dentistry* 13, no. 4 (2010): 265.

5. Julie Buring, lecture and slide presentation, T.H. Chan School of Public Health, Harvard University.

6. Chapter 8, "Case-Control and Cross Sectional Studies," in *Epidemiology for the Uninitiated*, The BMJ, https://www.bmj.com/about-bmj/resources-readers/publications/epidemiology-uninitiated/8-case-control-and-cross-sectional.

7. Buring, lecture and slide presentation.

8. Buring, lecture and slide presentation

9. Vinay Prasad and Vance W. Berger, "Hard-Wired Bias: How Even Double-Blind, Randomized Controlled Trials Can Be Skewed from the Start," *Mayo Clinic Proceedings* 90, no. 9 (2015): 1171–1175.

10. L. Talarico, G. Chen, and R. Pazdur, "Enrollment of Elderly Patients in Clinical Trials for Cancer Drug Registration: A 7-Year Experience by the US Food and Drug Administration," *Journal of Clinical Oncology* 22 (2004): 4626–4631.

11. Talal Hilal, Miguel Gonzalez-Velez, and Vinay Prasad, "Limitations in Clinical Trials Leading to Anticancer Drug Approvals by the US Food and Drug Administration," *JAMA Internal Medicine* 180, no. 8 (2020): 1108–1115.

12. James H. Ware and Mary Beth Hamel, "Pragmatic Trials—Guides to Better Patient Care," *New England Journal of Medicine* 364, no. 18 (2011): 1685–1687.

13. Heather Baer, lecture and slide presentation, T.H. Chan School of Public Health, Harvard University.

14. Kristine Broglio, "Randomization in Clinical Trials: Permuted Blocks and Stratification," *JAMA* 319, no. 21 (2018): 2223–2224.

15. Miguel Hernan, lecture and slide presentation, T.H. Chan School of Public Health, Harvard University.

16. Hernan, lecture and slide presentation.

Chapter 17. Catch Me If You Can

1. "Health Care Fraud and Abuse Control Program Report," HHS Office of Inspector General, https://oig.hhs.gov/reports-and-publications /hcfac/index.asp.

2. Lewis Morris, "Combating Fraud in Health Care: An Essential Component of Any Cost Containment Strategy," *Health Affairs* 28, no. 5 (2009): 1351–1356.

3. Jack Hadley and John Holahan, "How Much Medical Care Do the Uninsured Use, and Who Pays for It?," *Health Affairs* 22, Suppl. 1 (2003): W3–W66.

4. "Health Care Fraud," Cigna, https://www.cigna.com/reportfraud/.

5. Heather Landi, "Number of Patient Records Breached Nearly Triples in 2019," Fierce Healthcare, February 20, 2020, https://www.fiercehealthcare .com/tech/number-patient-records-breached-2019-almost-tripled-from-2018 -as-healthcare-faces-new-threats.

6. Landi, "Number of Patient Records."

7. Health Landi, "Healthcare Data Breaches Cost an Average $6.5M: Report," Fierce Healthcare, July 23, 2019, https://www.fiercehealthcare.com /tech/healthcare-data-breach-costs-average-6-45m-60-higher-than-other -industries-report.

8. Landi, "Healthcare Data Breaches."

9. Sammy Almashat, Sidney M. Wolfe, and Michael Carome, *Twenty-Five Years of Pharmaceutical Industry Criminal and Civil Penalties: 1991 through 2015* (Washington, DC: Public Citizen, March 31, 2016).

10. Angela Monaghan, "Pfizer Fined Record £84.2M over NHS Overcharging," *The Guardian*, December 6, 2016, https://www .theguardian.com/business/2016/dec/07/pfizer-fined-nhs-anti-epilepsy -drug-cma.

11. Ed Silverman, "Roche and Novartis Lose a Key Battle over Antitrust Fines in Italy," *STAT*, January 23, 2018, https://www.statnews.com /pharmalot/2018/01/23/roche-novartis-avastin-lucentis.

12. "Japan Files Criminal Complaint against Pharma Giant," World Finance, February 18, 2014, https://www.worldfinance.com/strategy/legal -management/japan-files-criminal-complaint-against-pharma-giant.

13. Jan Hoffman, "Opioid Settlement Offer Provokes Clash between States and Cities," *New York Times*, March 13, 2020, https://www.nytimes .com/2020/03/13/health/opioids-settlement.html.

14. Jan Hoffman, "Payout from a National Opioids Settlement Won't Be as Big as Hoped," *New York Times*, February 17, 2020, updated October 21, 2020, https://www.nytimes.com/2020/02/17/health/national-opioid -settlement.html.

15. Brian Fung, "Why It Took Facebook So Long to Act against the Doctored Pelosi Video," CNN, May 25, 2019, https://www.cnn.com/2019/05 /25/politics/facebook-pelosi-video-factchecking/index.html.

16. Sarah Frier, "Facing Lawmaker Questions, Says It May Remove Anti-Vaccine Recommendations," Facebook, February 14, 2019, https:// www.bloomberg.com/news/articles/2019-02-14/facebook-says-it-may -remove-anti-vaccine-recommendations.

17. Luiz Romero, "Roger Stone's Indictment Hints at the Origin of the #HillaryHealth Conspiracy Theories," Quartz, January 25, 2019, https://qz .com/1533847/roger-stones-indictment-reveals-plan-to-discredit-hillary -clintons-health/.

Chapter 18. Let Freedom Ring

1. Legal Information Institute, http://www.law.cornell.edu/constitu-tion/first_amendment; accessed May 2020.

2. Jeanie Kim and Amy Kapczynski, "Promotion of Drugs for Off-Label Uses: The US Food and Drug Administration at a Crossroads," *JAMA Internal Medicine* 177, no. 2 (2017): 157–158.

3. Brady Dennis, "FDA Has Free-Speech, Safety Issues to Weigh in Review of 'Off-Label' Drug Marketing Rules," *Washington Post*, July 9, 2014, http://www.washingtonpost.com/national/health-science/2014/07/09/3708dd6a-fbc4-11e3-8176-f2c941cf35f1_story.html.

4. Tim K. Mackey and Bryan A. Liang, "After *Amarin v FDA*: What Will the Future Hold for Off-Label Promotion Regulation?," *Mayo Clinic Proceed-ings* 91, no. 6 (2016): P701–P706.

5. D. C. Radley, S. N. Finkelstein, and R. S. Stafford, "Off-Label Prescribing among Office-Based Physicians," *Archives of Internal Medicine* 166, no. 9 (2006): 1021–1026.

6. C. M. Wittich, C. M. Burkle, and W. L. Lanier, "Ten Common Questions (and Their Answers) about Off-Label Drug Use," *Mayo Clinic Proceedings* 87, no. 10 (2012): 982–990.

7. Mackey and Liang, "After *Amarin v FDA*."

8. Kim and Kapczynski, "Promotion of Drugs for Off-Label Uses."

9. Margaret Wente, "We Can't Turn Doctors into Moral Eunuchs," *Globe and Mail*, August 7, 2014, https://www.theglobeandmail.com/opinion/we-cant-turn-doctors-into-moral-eunuchs/article19946476/.

10. Sarah C. Hull, "Not So Conscientious Objection: When Can Doctors Refuse to Treat," *STAT*, November 8, 2019, https://www.statnews.com/2019/11/08/conscientious-objection-doctors-refuse-treatment/.

11. Hull, "Not So Conscientious Objection."

Conclusion

1. Scott Mautz, "Warren Buffett's Little Known 'Noah Rule' Is the Key to Surviving Adversity," *Inc.*, accessed December 12, 2020, https://www.inc.com/scott-mautz/warren-buffetts-little-known-noah-rule-is-key-to-surviving-adversity.html.

INDEX

Abel, Thomas, 73
accountability and patient satisfaction, 39
actions, converting thought to, 193–95
acute care and patient satisfaction, 39
advertising, 113–14, 156–57
Affordable Care Act (ACA), 16–25
age: health expenditures by, 145–48; and invincibility complex, 115–16
Ahn, Ho-Young, 113–14
AI (artificial intelligence), 97, 98–107
Allergan, 6–8
Alzheimer's disease and optimism bias, 110–11
Amarin Pharma, Inc. v. FDA, 185, 187–88
American Medical Association, complaints to, 56–57
American Medical Collection Agency, 174–75
AmerisourceBergen, 178
Amerland, David, 99
analytic studies, understanding, 164–70
Anderson, Gerard, 5
artificial intelligence (AI), 97, 98–107
association *vs.* causation, 162–63, 171
Avastin, 176

Barzilay, Regina, 105–6
Bayes' theorem, 194
behavioral economics: and ACA, 17; defined, 17; impact of, 65–66; and ratings sites, 60. *See also* nudges
Bender, Eric, 105
Berk, Marc L., 143–44
Berkshire Hathaway, 193
Berle, Milton, 156
Bernoulli, Daniel, 68–69

bias: confounding, 49, 164, 169–70; and happiness, 35; lead-time bias, 96–97; optimism bias, 110–16; recall bias, 43; and screening programs, 95–97; selection bias, 35; in studies, 167; volunteer bias, 95–96
Bickert, Monika, 180
big data dilemma, 100
biological onset and screening programs, 89–90
black box syndrome, 105–7
blood pressure example of screening programs, 91–92, 95
Boulding, W., 41
Bresch, Heather, 4, 6
Bristol Myers Squibb, 14
broken arm example of screening programs, 92–94, 95
Brooks, Oliver, 124–25
Buffett, Warren, 193
burglary and optimism bias, 110–11

Canada: civil liberties in, 188–91; happiness in, 34; national identity, 24; and Restasis, 6–7; tying payments to patient satisfaction in, 38
cancer: delays in care from COVID-19, 119; heterogeneity of, 140; and optimism bias, 110, 113, 116; screening programs for, 88, 89, 90, 96–97; study concerns, 166–67
cannabis, medical, 128–38
Cardinal Health, 178
CareDash, 57
caregivers: and patient satisfaction, 39; unhappiness with health care system, 28
Carome, Michael, 157
Caronia, Alfred, 184–85
case-control studies, 164–65
case reports, 163
case series, 163